/01

MEDICINE
QUEST

VIKING
75 years

ALSO BY MARK J. PLOTKIN

Tales of a Shaman's Apprentice

The Shaman's Apprentice
(with Lynne Cherry)

Sustainable Marketing and Harvest
of Rain Forest Products
(edited with Lisa Famolare)

Mark J. Plotkin, Ph.D.

MEDICINE
QUEST

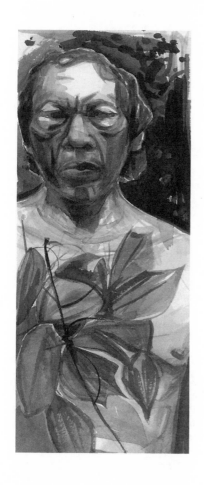

*In Search
of
Nature's
Healing
Secrets*

VIKING

VIKING
Published by the Penguin Group
Penguin Putnam Inc., 375 Hudson Street,
New York, New York 10014, U.S.A.
Penguin Books Ltd, 27 Wrights Lane, London W8 5TZ, England
Penguin Books Australia Ltd, Ringwood, Victoria, Australia
Penguin Books Canada Ltd, 10 Alcorn Avenue,
Toronto, Ontario, Canada M4V 3B2
Penguin Books (N.Z.) Ltd, 182–190 Wairau Road,
Auckland 10, New Zealand

Penguin Books Ltd, Registered Offices:
Harmondsworth, Middlesex, England

First published in 2000 by Viking Penguin,
a member of Penguin Putnam Inc.

3   5   7   9   10   8   6   4   2

Illustrations by Laurence Richardson
Page iii: Jaguar Shaman of the Tirio Indian tribe,
northeast Amazon

LIBRARY OF CONGRESS CATALOGING IN PUBLICATION DATA
Plotkin, Mark J.
Medicine quest : in search of
nature's healing secrets / Mark J. Plotkin
p.   cm.
Includes index.
ISBN 0-670-86937-6
1. Pharmacognosy Popular works.   I. Title.
RS160.P57   2000
615'.321—dc21   99-42822

This book is printed on acid-free paper.

Printed in the United States of America
Set in Aldus

For my beloved Liliana

ACKNOWLEDGMENTS

I am indebted to many people whose assistance, encouragement, insight, and experience made this book possible. My primary debt of gratitude is to my friends Dr. Adrian Forsyth and Rafe Sagalyn, who both suggested that I undertake this effort and who helped shape it along the way. I also wish to thank Dr. Paul Auerbach, Carolyn Carlson, Casey Fuetsch, Dr. Steve Grenard, Sy Montgomery, Dr. Gary Nabhan, Dr. David Newman, Michael Shnayerson, and Dr. Doug Steel for extraordinary editorial input.

I would like to express my appreciation to the following family, friends, colleagues, and organizations: Dr. Michael Adams, Akoi, Dr. Karriem Ali, Dr. Manuel Alonso, Dr. Stephen Altschul, the Amazon Conservation Team, the Arlington Public Library, Dr. Alan Attie, Dr. Silviano Camberos, Craig Canine, Virginia Cassell, Dr. Jack Cover, Dr. Gordon Cragg, Dr. John Daly, Dr. A. Der Marderosian, Dr. Jim Duke, Dr. Thomas Eisner, Dr. Terry Erwin, Lorena Espinoza, Dr. William Fenical, Dr. William Gerwick, Nicole Gibson, Dr. Jane Goodall, Peter Gorman, Dr. Robert Gould, Dr. Michael Goulding, Dr. Hugh Govan, Kate Griggs, Corinne Harpster, Chris Healy, Dr. Robert Heffron, Dr. Kathie Hodge, Bruce Hoffman, Dr. Michael Huffman, Dr. Bob Jacobs, Dr. Frank Keller, Ethan Kline, Dr. Robert Lazarus, Dr. Stuart Levy, Dr. Charles Limbach, Dr. Thomas Lovejoy, Loren McIntyre, Dr. Dennis McKenna, Liliana Madrigal, Victor Maldonado, Marion Maneker, Dr. Rob McCaleb, Dr. Donald McGraw, Dr. George Miljanich, Dr. Scott Mori, Sr. Luciano Mutumbajoy, Dr. Harriette Nadler, Nahtahlah, Dr. Ruth Noland, Mary O'Grady, Dr. Baldomero Olivera, Roland Ottewell, Ward and Mary Paine, Ann Lauren Plotkin, Gabrielle Plotkin, Helene Plotkin, Norman Plotkin, Dr. Shirley Pomponi, Henk and Judi Reichart, Dr. John Riddle, Becky Rose, Dr. Glenn Rothfield, Dr. Ethan Russo, Dr. Roy Sawyer, Dr. R. E. Schultes, Paula Sculley, Dr. Ronald Sherman, Dr. Shawn Sigstedt, David Stone, Dr. Tim Tankosic, Pam Trejos, Dr. Michael Tyler, Dr. R. Vander Meer, Dr. Marc van Roosmalen, Frits van Troon, Richard Wallace, Lucia Watson, Dr. Michael Williams, Dr. E. O. Wilson, Dr. Richard Wrangham, and Dr. German Zuluaga.

CONTENTS

INTRODUCTION

Nature distributed medicine everywhere.
—Pliny the Elder, circa A.D. 77

I can vividly recall the mixture of horror and fascination I felt more than forty years ago as I sat on the linoleum floor of my beloved grandmother's kitchen in Plaquemine, Louisiana, watching her inject herself with insulin to combat the dreaded diabetes that had killed so many family members back in the old country. The insulin kept the disease under control for many decades, but about fifteen years ago her body began to reject it—as is so often the case—and her inexorable decline commenced. Her bright and cheerful nature gave way to a persistent listlessness, and her eyesight began to fail. She developed gangrene in both feet that slowly spread into her legs. The doctor amputated both limbs, but to no avail. Her deterioration was slow and painful, and powerful painkillers provided minimal relief. The disease killed her two years later.

So it was with some distress, sitting in a little thatch hut deep in the forest of the northeast Amazon, that I explained the illness, and my desire to find new treatments for it, to the paramount shamans of the Tirio Indian tribe. My plea for assistance was met by a moment of silence, and then the shamans conferred quietly among themselves. Finally, my old mentor, the Jaguar Shaman, spoke on behalf of the group: "My son, we do not know this disease that you describe. We do not have a name for it, do not recognize the symptoms as you describe them, do not have plants to treat it. Perhaps the disease exists, but we do not know it. We are sorry we cannot help you."

I was discouraged but not surprised. As an ethnobotanist, a scientist who works with indigenous peoples to document their uses of local plants, I'd been studying the healing practices of the shamans of the northeast Amazon for almost fifteen years. With the Tirios (the original Amazon warriors), I'd hunted forest pigs with poison-tipped arrows; with the Akuriyos (a tribe of semi-nomadic hunter-gatherers), I'd found plants that could cure excruciating insect stings within minutes; and with the Yanomami (the so-called Fierce People), I'd participated in curing rituals that entailed the ingestion of titanic quantities of hallucinogenic snuff. Yet in twelve years of working with the Tirio tribe, I had never seen a case of diabetes (at least one that I could recognize). I turned to the physician who had been sent with me to provide Western health care to the villagers and to assist me with my research. "We should pack up and get ready to move out on the cargo plane that'll be here next week," I said.

He nodded his assent, replying, "That will give me plenty of time to finish seeing everyone who needs my help."

The next morning was so exceedingly hot I was sweating before I woke up. As I sat up rubbing the sleep out of my eyes, I was visited by an old friend from a neighboring tribe. Akoi was a Sikiyana-Chikena, a people famed for their bellicose nature, the "dread and terror of their more peaceable neighbors," according to an early explorer's account. Their traditional homelands lay to the southwest, along the banks of the mighty Trombetas River. We exchanged greetings in Portuguese, which we both spoke well enough to converse freely. I began conveying my disappointment that I had come so far in search of a treatment for diabetes, yet the Tirios appeared to know neither the disease nor a remedy for it.

He was unfamiliar with the term "diabetes." "Describe the symptoms," he said.

I told him about the sores between the toes, the incessant thirst, the fading eyesight.

His face broke into a triumphant smile. "Well, maybe the Tirios don't know that sickness, but I do!" he said.

Stunned, I asked him, "You know this ailment?"

"Sure!" he said.

"C-can you treat it?" I stammered.

"Of course!" he replied, confidently. "Come on, I'll show you how." I grabbed my machete and followed him to the edge of the village where the jungle began. Together we entered the twilight-green world of the forest. First he used his machete to peel long strips of white bark off a towering tree and then scraped the pinkish red inner bark onto the cut leaf of a wild banana. Then he added the crushed waxy green leaves of a trailside herb to the pile. Next he sliced off the stems of a twisted gray vine that snaked its way into the canopy, and he carefully collected the sap into a container he made from the leaf of a nearby palm. We brought it all back to the village; I measured and weighed each ingredient to get the precise recipe before the old shaman began boiling it all together in an ancient clay pot over a wood fire.

As he stirred the potion, I began writing a detailed account of the experience in my field notebook. A firm believer in checking, checking, and rechecking information (especially when working in a second language), I asked him to describe the symptoms of the disease he treated with the medicine he was busily preparing.

"You wash with it when you are unable to urinate," he said, "and you drink it when your feet are sore."

I was stunned. Clearly, this was not a treatment for diabetes. Had something been lost in translation? Had he shown me this remedy merely out of a desire to please or impress me? Or was this perhaps some sort of trick to humiliate or test me? Not knowing the answers, I was uncertain how to proceed. I re-asked the question about which affliction could be treated by the potion and received the same response. The shaman finally said that the potion was ready and I filled two plastic sample jars with the thick reddish brown liquid. I thanked the shaman and, confused and a bit crestfallen, carried the bottles through a tropical downpour back to my thatched hut.

That night, I was writing up my field notes by the dim yellow light of a kerosene lantern on a makeshift wooden table while the physician accompanying me saw his patients in the back of the hut. He came out suddenly, clearly shaken. "Come quickly!" he said. "You have to see this!"

His agitation was palpable. I picked up my lantern and ducked into his little examining room. Stretched out on an ancient dusty cot lay a woman dying of diabetes. She was about thirty-five, pale, bloated, nauseated, and weak, with persistent itching in her legs. She had a burning thirst and gangrenous sores between several of her toes.

"That's it," he said excitedly, "classic type 2 diabetes! I've taken a blood-sugar level reading and it's over five hundred, almost fatal."

"What can you do for her? What'll you give her?" I asked.

"You tell me," he replied. "We're in the middle of the jungle here. Even if I had insulin, there's no way to keep it chilled so it won't spoil. I had some pills that can temporarily reduce blood sugar, but I ran out of those on my last expedition and forgot to buy more. Besides, what would I have done with insulin? Shoot her full of it and then leave her to die?"

Just then, as if by some sort of jungle magic, the Sikiyana healer appeared at the entrance to our hut. He entered and looked over the patient, asked her a few questions, did a brief examination, and turned to me, saying, "That's the disease I was telling you about. What are you going to give her?"

We admitted that we had no medicine that would effectively treat her condition.

"Where's the potion I made for you today?" I handed him one of the bottles and he unscrewed the top. He asked the physician for a spoon, filled it twice, and gave it to his patient, then helped her back to her hut. By the next morning, her blood-sugar level was almost normal. The Sikiyana continued to give her the medicine four times a day; within three days, she felt well enough to return to working in her garden, something she'd been unable to do for two years. By the end of the week, her blood-sugar level was normal and the gangrenous sore that had oozed between her toes for over eighteen months had started to heal.

·   ·   ·

For almost twenty years I've been combing the remote corners of the Amazon jungle searching for plants that heal. I am an ethnobotanist—a plant hunter, a shaman's apprentice—on the trail of natural compounds that can treat diseases for which modern medicine has no cure. For all those involved—ethnobotanists, marine biologists, chemists, physicians, even rain forest shamans—this is a quest powered by the desperation of the ill and the compassion of those who would cure them.

As our culture races to embrace technology, it may seem quaint or quixotic to seek new therapeutic compounds from the world around us. Yet the history of Western civilization can be written in terms of its reliance on and utilization of natural products. Western medicine still depends on plants and animals—our hospitals, pharmacies, and medicine chests brim with drugs derived from nature.

While the invention of synthetic chemistry in the 1930s reduced our reliance on the natural world as our sole source of medicines, an electrifying renaissance is well under way as we comb the far corners of the planet for healing compounds. Within the course of the past decade, this quest has gone from being a marginal exercise to a mainstream concern. Mother Nature has been devising extraordinary chemicals for more than 3.5 billion years, and new technologies increasingly facilitate our ability to discover, study, manipulate, and use these compounds as never before. The best evidence: during the last five years, most major pharmaceutical companies have launched new programs to find, isolate, analyze, and develop these medicines. *New technologies enhance, rather than diminish, nature's value as a source of healing compounds.*

At the dawn of the twenty-first century, scientists hang by slender nylon ropes in rain forest canopies 120 feet above the forest floor, collecting undocumented species of spiders whose venom could revolutionize the way we treat chronic pain and paralysis. Meanwhile, other researchers don dry suits and dive below the polar ice caps to capture fish that have evolved a natural antifreeze that may one day improve the way we store organs to be transplanted. And still others trek across burning desert sands, searching for vipers whose poison may help reinvent the treatment of high blood pressure. The hunt for nature's healing magic represents an eternal quest that has taken us into the tombs of the pharaohs, the gleaming futuristic laboratories of the National Institutes of Health, and the recently discovered hydrothermal vents in jagged cracks and crevasses that furrow the ocean's floor. This book details that search—past, present, and future—as we follow in the footsteps of those who have sought, and continue to seek, miraculous new medicines from Mother Nature.

Chapter One

SOME POISON FOR YOUR PAIN?

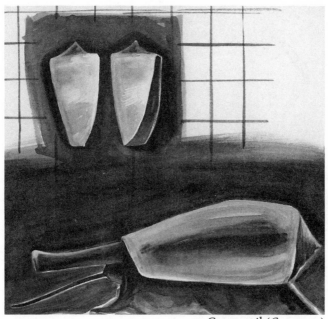

Cone snail (*Conus sp.*)

The difference between a deadly poison and a life-saving medicine can be very small; in fact, it is sometimes merely a question of dosage.

—Dr. R. E. Schultes, 1980

Time was running out, and the indefatigable frog detective Dr. John Daly decided to risk everything in one of the boldest scientific crapshoots of the twentieth century.

Daly had in his possession a tiny vial of an almost irreplaceable frog-skin extract that held the possibility of revolutionizing the way we treat pain, that might be turned into a billion-dollar-a-year medicine, and that might relieve incredible agony and human suffering. Yet he knew that analyzing the compound would destroy what little he had left of the precious substance, and he was fully aware that he might not ever be able to find it again.

For over a quarter century, Daly had been combing the most remote jungles of Central and South America, braving bandits, guerrillas, narcotraffickers, malaria, and myriad other hazards on what many would consider to be a quixotic quest: he was in search of tiny poison dart frogs and the powerful chemicals embedded in their skin. Daly knew that Indians in northwestern Colombia rubbed the skins of these frogs on their blowdarts so that even a scratch would prove lethal. He had already found a one-inch species—the aptly named *Phyllobates terribilis*—a single individual of which harbored enough poison to kill ten men or twenty thousand mice. It was Daly's fervent belief that these potent poisons might one day help alleviate human suffering.

When Daly began his investigations in the 1960s, the technology necessary to analyze the frog compounds was both slow and tedious. Unlike the Amazonian *cururu* frog, which can tip the scales at over seven pounds, poison arrow frogs are tiny enough to perch comfortably on the tip of your little finger. Not only was Daly sometimes unable to collect enough frogs to extract the amounts necessary to complete the study, but the chemical complexity of these compounds made it nearly impossible to synthesize them in the lab.

A 1966 article on Daly's research on Colombian frogs was published in *Medical World News* and caught the eye of Charles Myers, then a graduate student conducting research in Panama and now a senior scientist at the American Museum of Natural History in New York City. Unlike Daly, who was primarily trained as a chemist, Myers was a herpetologist, a biologist specializing in reptiles and amphibians, hence his background complemented that of Daly's. Myers wrote a letter to Daly proposing a collaboration that has continued to the present day.

The two Americans began their collaboration in Panama but then moved south. In 1974, they collected a brilliantly colored orange, red, and white frog known as *Epipedobates tricolor* near Santa Isabel in southwestern Ecuador. When Daly injected an extract of *Epipedobates* skin into a mouse, the rodent immediately arched its tail over its back, the so-called Straub tail reaction, which is the response usually generated by an opium-like painkiller. Believing he had found merely an amphibian equivalent of opium, the scientist then treated the mouse with naloxone, an opiate blocker, which he expected would cause the creature to lower its tail. The mouse, however, did not respond and the tail remained arched over its back. This intrigued and excited Daly because it meant that he was on the trail of one of the Holy Grails of modern medicine: a nonsedating, potentially nonaddictive, nonopioid painkiller. Not only did the new chemical—named "epibatidine" in honor of the frog—kill pain, but it also proved two hundred times more potent than morphine and it appeared to exert its effects in a manner completely different from that of opium.

The bad news, however, was that epibatidine was too toxic and had too many negative side effects to be used on humans. Daly and his colleagues thought they might analyze the molecule to determine its exact structure, which would allow them to manipulate the epibatidine molecule in order to produce a version less toxic but still potent. Unfortunately, the laboratory technology necessary for purifying, analyzing, and synthesizing the molecule did not exist at the time. And they had used up the little bit of poison they had managed to collect. It was time to return to the jungle.

The original epibatidine had been extracted from frogs collected from two different locales in 1974. When the scientists returned to Ecuador two years later, one population of the amphibians had completely vanished; much of the surrounding forest had been felled and converted to banana plantations. Fortunately, they were able to find these frogs at the other site—but only enough to collect less than one milligram of the poison! Then, in 1984, passage of the Convention on International Trade in Endangered Species (CITES) Treaty made it exceedingly difficult (if not impossible) to legally collect and export poison dart frogs, particularly in the large quantities necessary for chemical analysis of the toxin. And habitat destruction in western Ecuador was on the increase. Attempts to breed the frogs in the lab were successful, but the frogs contained no epibatidine! So Daly had a tiny and finite supply of epibatidine and demand for the compound for testing purposes was increasing. Daly stored his precious poison, awaiting the day when modern technology would improve to the point of being able to unlock one of Mother Nature's most closely guarded (and potentially useful) secrets.

In 1990, Daly decided it was time to roll the dice. Out of his freezer he took the tiny vial with the precious epibatidine inside. No new epibatidine had been collected in more than a decade. Meanwhile, the frogs' habitat was being decimated as the human population in southwestern Ecuador greatly expanded, causing an enormous decline in forest cover. However, analytical methods and instruments had greatly improved with tools like nuclear magnetic resonance (NMR) and gas chromatography-infrared spectroscopy, made all the more effective by the microchip revolution already well under way. Since the analysis of the chemical entailed the destruction of the tiny sample that Daly had, the decision to analyze the epibatidine was an enormous gamble.

The gamble paid off: the structure of the molecule was revealed. Within two years, scientists were able to synthesize the molecule to create a limitless supply for experimentation. Laboratories around the world eagerly began investigating the potential utility of this strange chemical from a tiny rain forest frog.

Interestingly, epibatidine bears a chemical resemblance to nicotine. Right around the time that Daly and his colleagues were determining the chemical structure of epibatidine, researchers at Abbott Laboratories were investigating nicotine-like chemicals for the treatment of Alzheimer's disease. Taking note of the similar structure of epibatidine, but aware that it was too toxic for human use, they began to create similar compounds, hoping that one might prove highly effective as a painkiller. Of the hundreds of molecules devised and tested, one stood out: ABT-594. Not only did it lack the toxicity of epibatidine, but it proved effective against several types of pain, including one caused by nerve damage against which even opiates are relatively ineffective. Unlike opiates, ABT-594 appears to be nonaddictive, enhances alertness rather than causing sedation, and has relatively little effect on the respiratory system.

Because it is so different from morphine, it appears to offer unlimited potential as a treatment for pain, provided that epibatidine makes it through the FDA approval process and enters the marketplace. Dr. Michael Williams of Abbott Labs stated, "It lacks the major side effects of morphine like constipation and addiction. ABT-594 is proving to be a very interesting molecule."

It is the fervent belief of scientists like Daly and Williams that these and other potent natural poisons will help alleviate human suffering.

A poison is any substance—man-made or found in nature—that produces disease conditions, tissue injury, or otherwise interrupts natural life processes when in contact with the body. Toxins are poisonous substances produced by living creatures, including amphibians, bacteria, insects, plants, and reptiles. Venoms are poisons of animal origin that are injected by spines (such as is the case with sea urchins), stings (such as honeybees), or teeth (rattlesnakes). Poisonous creatures have always been objects of fear and fascination. People worshiped deadly cobras in ancient India. The bite of the tarantula was believed by denizens of Europe in the Middle Ages to cause an uncontrollable urge to dance (the whirling folk dance known as the "tarantella" was inspired by this notion). And citizens of the American South still handle venomous serpents to demonstrate their devotion to the Lord.

But these days it is the major pharmaceutical companies that are most interested in these poisons, and the stakes are huge: a single blockbuster drug (like the high-blood-pressure drug Capoten, which was developed based on studies of Brazilian viper venom) can earn over 1.5 billion dollars per year.

The Holy Grail of current drug study is finding a new medicament that is effective for treating a particular malady (particularly an ailment that has no other effective treatment or cure) and which meets certain criteria. The compound should ideally have a unique and (previously) unknown chemical structure (making it easier to patent); function in a unique pathway in the human body (meaning that it operates differently and, we hope, more effectively than other pharmaceuticals used to treat a given condition); be a small molecule (making it easier and less expensive to synthesize); be quick acting; and have no unwanted side effects (such as addiction, for example).

Venoms are the end result of billions of years of evolution. These molecules have been honed to generate a response in the body of the victim that is quick, dramatic, and often fatal. This response may include pain, numbness, asphyxiation, hemorrhage, clotting, shock, paralysis, or a change in blood pressure. Some venoms are composed of hundreds of various poisons, each of which does something different when injected into the body of another creature. Precisely because these poisons are so refined, their potential as medicines is enormous.

For example, eriostatin, a protein from an Asian pit viper, appears to inhibit the spread of melanoma cells, and a compound based on the venom of an Israeli scorpion binds to the cells of a type of brain cancer and seems to keep them from spreading to other parts of the body. SNX-482, from Cameroon red tarantula venom, may lead to a new class of medicines for the treatment of neurological disorders. Gila monsters from the American Southwest have a substance in their venom known as exendin, which stimulates the secretion of insulin, meaning it may one day be used to prevent the progression of diabetes. And an enzyme in the venom of the Russell's pit viper, one of the world's most beautiful and most deadly snakes, is now being employed in a diagnostic test for lupus.

Toxins produced by lethal organisms are also being employed for medical uses. Minuscule amounts of the deadly botulism bacteria are proving to be effective for the treatment of a rare condition that paralyzes the vocal cords. Under the trade name Botox, botulism toxin is being injected into facial muscles that cause wrinkles. The toxin temporarily paralyzes them, resulting in a surgeryless face-lift (though given the choice between surgery and having one of the world's most poisonous substances injected into their heads, most people still choose the knife).

Toxin molecules typically accomplish their deadly tasks through a three-stage process: first they attach to a healthy cell, then they enter the cell, and then they exert their deadly effects on the cell's machinery, causing it to malfunction and/or die. Working with a form of the deadly diphtheria bacillus, scientists are devising the means to deliver a poison into cancer cells, thereby destroying them. Similar efforts are under way with the tetanus toxin to treat diseases like Tay-Sachs.

Venoms continue to play an absolutely fundamental role in our understanding of how cells function. They have proven essential in helping us comprehend ion channels, which are pores on a cell's surface that control the flow of calcium, potassium, and sodium in and out of the cells, and which play a key role in transmission of nerve impulses (that is, how nerve cells talk to and activate each other). Because these venoms are highly specific and only interact with particular channels, they are of inestimable use in mapping these channels. In the words of the National Cancer Institute's Dr.

David Newman: "Using venoms, we can turn something on—or off—in a particular cell which teaches you something about the function of that cell. You can block a certain response and observe what happens when you add something like a medicine. You can learn about everything from the structure and function of ion channels to how cells communicate with each other."

In the laboratory, venoms help teach us how medicines function in the human body. Drugs tend to operate in two basic ways. Many interact directly with the body's metabolism. Aspirin represents a classic example, mitigating pain by interfering with the body's production of prostaglandins, which cause the discomfort. Other drugs attack or interfere with the disease-causing organism itself. Penicillin would fall into this category—it inhibits the ability of the invading bacteria's cells to reproduce but does not interact with human cells.

All drugs have a "target" (a site of action) in the body. Many of these targets are receptors, protein molecules on the cell's surface that interact with other molecules. (The receptor is often described as the lock into which the "key" molecule must fit.) Drugs can either fit into receptors and elicit a certain response (in which case they are termed "agonists") or they can block the receptors, eliciting no response but keeping other chemical messengers from interacting with the receptors ("antagonists").

As with the ion channels, some venom components interact only with very specific receptors, allowing us to map our nervous systems in extraordinary detail. Knowledge of these receptor sites is already helping scientists to design some drugs from scratch. In the future, when all the receptor sites on all the cells have been mapped, scientists may design all drugs that way. Until that day, however, Mother Nature will play an essential role.

Though venoms are being investigated as the source of new treatments for everything from cancer to diabetes, they are probably most promising as sources of pain relievers. Many venomous animals use poison as a means of trapping their prey rather than as a defense against enemies. How? By immobilizing it so it cannot fight or flee! The most effective way to achieve this is to interfere with—or shut down—the prey's nervous system. And, for our own treatment purposes, we are learning how to use some of venom's unique properties to close down only a certain part of the nervous system, and hence block pain.

Pain represents the most common reason people visit their physicians, and chronic pain is an oft-stated reason that severely ill people give when they ask their physicians' assistance in committing suicide. Pain is usually caused by burns, cuts, pricks, excessive pressure, or other factors telling us that our body is being damaged. The very few people born with the inability to feel pain often suffer terribly for it, not realizing, until the damage is already done, that the water they stuck their hand into is too hot or that the knife they are using to slice an onion has just cut deeply into their finger.

In other cases, a problem occurs when the brain continues to receive pain messages even after the causative agent has ceased inflicting the pain. In the case of "phantom limb syndrome," the limb continues to "hurt" years after it has been amputated. This pain presumably results from crossed signals in the brain (or crossed signals in nerves near the amputated limb) rather than damage to a limb that is no longer there. Naturally, this offers little solace to the three million Americans who suffer from this malady.

The amount of such "incurable" suffering that a new natural drug might relieve is staggering in terms of both numbers and dollars. According to the *New York Times*, between thirty million and eighty million Americans suffer from pain ineffectively treated by common analgesics (painkillers). At least six million experience pain caused by damaged nerves; another million suffer excruciating pain due to various cancers; while still others are subjected to suffering caused by everything from AIDS to spinal cord injuries. At least one study has suggested that the annual cost of medical bills and lost wages due to pain is as high as one hundred billion dollars. The annual retail value of morphine and morphine-derived products in this country is about six hundred million dollars.

Exceedingly promising as sources of new venom-derived painkillers and other powerful potions are the aquatic masters of immobilization: the cone snails of the tropical coral reefs. Dr. Newman of the National Cancer Institute has called them "for their size, the deadliest creatures on our planet." Cone snails are the archers of the deep: they kill by shooting their prey with an arrow. The arrows are actually the snail's teeth, which are contained inside a long tube that is the "tongue" of the creature and is longer than the snail's body. Each arrow is a hollow and disposable harpoon and contains a deadly poison. The cone snails not only developed this type of hunting long before we did, they also invented the disposable syringe in the process! The case of Steve C. demonstrates the medical potential of cone snails:

Steve's medical problems began at an age when most kids have little more on their minds than whom to play with in their kindergarten class. At the age of five, several of the toes on his left foot began to ache, the result of a rare form of cancer that started there and spread throughout the rest of his body. As if cancer invading the soft tissues of his body wasn't enough of a curse, the disease caused unbearable pain that sometimes reduced him to writhing on the floor on the verge of unconsciousness. Steve said, "It [was] as if somebody stabs you and twists the knife . . . it would go on sometimes for hours."

To relieve his misery, Steve relied on the best Western medicine for treating intractable pain: opium and opiate derivatives, which have been valued for their analgesic effects by humankind for thousands of years. He took morphine pills and applied synthetic morphine patches. Other narcotics were added to the mix when these powerful compounds didn't do the job. But morphine and the synthetic and semisynthetic compounds based on it cause serious side effects like addiction, constipation, and respiratory distress. Most problematic from the standpoint of someone suffering intolerable pain, the body grows accustomed to the drug so that, over time, more of it is needed to obtain relief. Some pain sufferers must take over one hundred times the lethal dose of morphine just to make it through the day.

On the other side of the planet from where Steve grew up in the American Midwest, Baldomero "Toto" Olivera enjoyed a carefree bucolic boyhood near Manila. On weekends and holidays, the

entire family would travel by small seaplane to the Philippine island of Alabat, where they had a cottage that looked out over the
ocean. In 1942, when the Japanese invaded and captured Manila,
Toto's family fled to the island bungalow that they felt would be a
safe refuge in which to wait out the war.

Disappointed that he had to leave both his friends and most of
his toys behind, Toto developed a new hobby: collecting seashells.
He spent long afternoons walking along the sandy beaches amidst
the coconut palms, watching the waves break over the coral atolls
that encircled the island. The boy would stop to pick up seashells to
add to his burgeoning collection. But he never forgot the one type
of shell—the most beautiful of them all—that he was told harbored
a creature with a poisonous sting: the exquisitely mottled tapering
shell of the cone snail.

Cone snail shells have long been an obsession of collectors
around the world. Names given to each species—the Majestic
Cone, or the Glory of the Sea—only hint at their ethereal beauty.
How valuable are they? In 1796, a two-inch shell was auctioned
along with a painting by the Dutch master Vermeer: the snail shell
sold for seven times the purchase price of the painting.

Admiring their beauty, one has no sense of the poisons hidden
within. At least two species of these tiny creatures are capable of
killing a human being. Several years ago, a man snorkeling in the
Philippines happened upon a cone snail slowly making its way
along the coral reef. He picked it up and, not having a bag to put it
into, he stuffed it down the front of his bathing suit.

This is the kind of mistake you only make once.

Cone snails are great poison producers by necessity. Inside
their shells, they are essentially soft-bodied creatures. They cannot
afford to get into wrestling matches or tug-of-wars with every animal they want to eat—it might tear them apart. Consequently,
they have evolved fast-acting poisons that can kill their prey almost instantaneously. Some of their means of delivering the poison
verge on the ghoulish. One species of cone snail extends a proboscis
that looks like a piece of bait. As the fish approaches, expecting a
meal, it quickly becomes one instead. The snail shoots a poison-

tipped harpoon into the fish's mouth, instantly killing the fish, which is then quickly devoured.

After completing a Ph.D. in chemistry at Caltech, Toto returned to the Philippines anxious to use his newfound training to help his native land. His lab at the university had little sophisticated equipment, and even less of a research budget. Toto decided to look for a project that would focus on local resources, since he lacked the funding for a project that required international travel. Remembering the cone snails, he made a few inquiries and was surprised to learn that hardly any research had been done to determine the chemical composition of the poison. And virtually nothing had been done to evaluate whether it had any commercial or therapeutic potential.

Toto hypothesized that the venom contained a single toxic component. He was surprised when his initial investigations indicated the presence of at least nine different poisons. Moreover, the poisons had a unique composition and shape, comprising a new type of compound which Toto christened "conotoxins." But his cone snail research languished when Toto accepted a teaching position in Salt Lake City, far from the coral reefs that offered a ready supply of cone snails and their conotoxins. It was in Salt Lake, however, that an iconoclastic undergraduate named Craig Clark, searching for a research project topic, asked a simple question that eventually proved to have dazzling implications.

"Professor Olivera," he asked, "what would happen if we introduced single conotoxins directly into the mouse brain?"

"The mice would die," Toto replied. "Better not to waste your time and my mice. Can't you find another project?"

The student decided to give it a try anyway. The result? Rodent bedlam. The mice that received one compound began dancing frantically, while recipients of another began dragging their hind legs, while others scratched themselves or started swinging their heads from side to side. It was immediately obvious that each compound had a very different and very pronounced effect on the nervous system. Further research revealed that one of these conotoxins could disrupt the ability of nerve cells to communicate with each other. If this compound could be demonstrated to interrupt pain signals as they traveled from the human spinal cord to the brain, it would represent a new painkiller that might be used in addition to—or instead of—morphine.

That is exactly what Toto and his colleagues have found in one particular conotoxin. Initially known as MVIIB (and now called ziconotide), this compound attaches itself solely to a part of the spinal cord known as the dorsal horn, through which pass the nerve cells that convey pain signals from the body to the brain.

Dr. George Miljanich, chief chemist at Neurex/Elan, the company that is commercializing the compound, said, "[The drug] works by blocking proteins in the nervous system called calcium channels [that are] required for synaptic transmission, that is, for the nerve cells to talk to each other and activate each other. By blocking calcium channels and suppressing synaptic activity, the system is suppressed, its activity is lowered, and many physiological effects can ensue from that."

Steve C. takes ziconotide on a daily basis and has found it so effective that he no longer takes morphine. In fact, he sleeps comfortably through the night for the first time in over two decades. And other pain sufferers have responded equally well to the still experimental new drug. Some patients, completely bedridden and mentally addled by their use of morphine, switched to ziconotide and were able to leave the hospital and resume living a normal life.

Ziconotide is considered hundreds of times more potent than morphine; it offers three major advantages over morphine and other opiate-derived drugs. First, it has proven effective in treating pain (like the phantom limb syndrome or neuropathic pain) that cannot be relieved with other drugs. Second, the human body appears not to develop tolerance to the drug. Third, it is not addictive. If and when ziconotide is approved for general use and enters the marketplace, its nonaddictive effectiveness promises a potential annual retail value as high as one billion dollars per year.

Of course, not all promising leads result in new drugs. Current estimates are that only one of every ten thousand molecules that are investigated ever makes it into the pharmacy, the hospital, or the medicine chest. A recent issue of the *Economist* explained,

> Substances emerging from [an] initial screening (now usually carried out in a tissue culture rather than an animal) are rarely powerful enough to be effective as they stand. The next step, therefore, is for chemists to fiddle with the exact arrangement of a promising compound's atoms . . . in order to increase its potency [or decrease its toxicity, or both]. . . . The "lead compound" which results from this tinkering is then subjected to further tests, this time generally in animals. These show how well it is absorbed by the body, how it stands up to the biochemical rigours it meets there, how poisonous it is, and what sort of side effects it might be expected to produce. Only then is it allowed to go into clinical trials in people—first small ones to test its safety, and then much larger ones to prove its effectiveness for its intended job. If, after going through all this, the company thinks that it has a winner, it still has to persuade the regulatory authorities to agree. Only when a molecule has passed this final test does it pop out of the other end of the pipeline and on to the revenue line of the company's accounts.

This Food and Drug Administration (FDA) approval process consists of three separate phases. Phase 1 is comprised of safety trials in which low doses of the drug are given to just a few volunteers. The test subjects are monitored for harmful side effects over the course of several months. The next phase examines the effectiveness and safety of the drug in a small number of patients (up to several hundred) suffering from the disease in question. Phase 2 can take (on average) up to two years. In phase 3, however, the efficacy and safety of the drug is tested on a large patient population over the course of two to four years. If the results are positive, the pharmaceutical company files a New Drug Approval (NDA) request that is then usually approved by the FDA after the agency has reviewed the results, a process that takes about a year and a half. ABT-594, the poison dart frog derivative, is currently in phase 1, while ziconotide is in phase 3.

Perhaps the most exciting aspect of the cone snail research is that it currently entails much more than ziconotide. Each species may produce up to two hundred different venoms—and there are five hundred species of cone snails. According to Toto, some venomous creatures, like sea snakes, produce venoms that contain only one paralytic agent, most assuredly not the case with cone snails. Toto Olivera said, "The cone snail's poison wallops its prey with a speedball that kills the fish on impact. It is like being hit with Amazonian arrow poison, botulism toxin, puffer fish poison and the shock of an electric eel all at once."

The upshot of having and studying these thousands of powerful chemicals is that their therapeutic potential is by no means limited to pain. A 1990 article in the *Economist*, suitably entitled "Skip the Escargots," noted: "At least part of the problem in some neurological and psychiatric diseases is that ion channels or receptors are stimulated too much or too little. If the receptor at fault in a particular condition is identified, a drug could be made with a molecule based on the conotoxin design. It would react only with that receptor and so would not trigger any of the side-effects that come with many of the existing, unselective psychiatric drugs."

Toto recently parted ways with the firm that is commercializing ziconotide to help start another company. "There are about five hundred species of cone snails," he told me, "and each species may produce two hundred different poisons. If you take out ziconotide, you still have nine thousand nine hundred and ninety-nine compounds left to study. And others that I am already investigating have the potential to do for epilepsy and other central nervous system disorders what ziconotide does for pain."

Yet poison dart frogs, cone snails, and many other species are disappearing faster than we can study them. Wild populations of the Ecuadorean dart frog that led to the development of ABT-594 continue to dwindle. The *okopipi*, a brilliant blue dart frog found only on a few tiny forest islands surrounded by grasslands in the northeast Amazon, is being threatened by unscrupulous wildlife dealers who illegally collect them for export. Another species was almost wiped out on the Panamanian island of Taboga by a German reptile dealer. And cone snails live on coral reefs, one of the world's most threatened ecosystems. How much has already been lost, and what medical miracles have been sacrificed as a result?

Chapter Two

THE ETERNAL QUEST

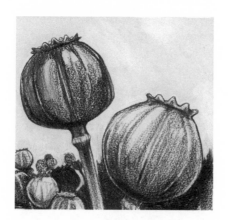

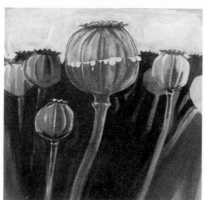

Opium poppies (*Papaver somniferum*)

*All we have yet discovered is but a trifle in comparison
with what still lies hid in the great treasury of Nature.*

—Anton von Leeuwenhoek, 1679

Scientists the world over are once again embarking on a medicine quest in search of new healing compounds from the world around us. It is a quest older than the written word: the earliest writings of all ancient civilizations brim with references to healing compounds, indicating a long history of experimentation with natural substances. The search for new medicines played an integral role in the Age of Discovery. Columbus was obsessed with spices, yet what we now employ mostly as condiments were once valued at least as highly for their medicinal value as their culinary appeal. Shortly after Cortés's conquest of the Aztecs, the king of Spain dispatched his court physician Hernandez to study, document, and retrieve the medicines of these Indians. Fusee Aublet, one of the first biologists to work in the Amazon, was sent to South America as "Apothecary-Botanist to the King of France."

The quest for healing may even predate our own species. It was once believed that humans were the only species that used medicine. No longer. At Shanidar Cave in Iraq, the skeleton of a Neanderthal was found buried with seven medicinal species of plants placed in a ring around the body. Both chimpanzees and gorillas employ plants for medicinal purposes, which implies that common ancestors we shared over a million years ago probably utilized plants for similar reasons. And we have recently learned that many animals—from dogs to coatimundis, from elephants to lemurs—rely on medicinal species. Not only does this demonstrate our commonality with other species, but it also points us in the direction of new healing compounds in the process.

The argument for preserving species solely for the medicines they can provide is, in a sense, selfish and shortsighted. Conservation of nature should be considered, in my opinion, a spiritual belief and ethical practice, and we should not decimate or extinguish species because of ignorance or greed. That said, however, the medical argument for conservation is still the most appealing and convincing justification we have for conservation, and one that can be understood by every member of our own species, regardless of nationality, political affiliation, or economic class. To understand how great an impact our study of nature will have on our lives (in the even relatively short-term future) in terms of medicine, we must consider the fact that several new blockbuster drugs derived from natural sources will hit the market in the course of the next decade. Synthetic drugs will continue to play a major role in the marketplace, but natural and semisynthetic medicines (based on chemicals that occur in nature that have been manipulated or duplicated in the lab) will increase in importance for the foreseeable future.

It is also essential to note that nature can contribute far more to healing than new wonder drugs. Nature plays a healing role in most human lives as the basis for aesthetic and spiritual inspiration. And a rapidly evolving science recently labeled "biomimicry" studies nature as a source of wisdom that can teach us everything from how to clean up industrial messes to how to create adhesives that hold their grip underwater. Harvard geneticist Dr. Richard Lewontin notes, "The one point I think all evolutionary biologists are agreed upon [is that] it is virtually impossible to do a better job than an organism is [already] doing in its own environment."

An oft-cited example of learning from nature is that of the Wright brothers, who began to understand the concepts of lift and drag by studying the flight of vultures. Currently, the pressure-resistant shell structure of ocean-dwelling snails is being studied by engineers to learn how to design better ceramics, concrete, and computer disks. In the words of the esteemed entomologist Dr. E. O. Wilson: "Each species is an evolutionary masterpiece."

Jeannine Benyus eloquently summed up the revolutionary potential of learning from other creatures in her book *Biomimicry:* "[Since the first organisms appeared almost four billion years ago] . . . life has learned to fly, circumnavigate the globe, live in the depths of the ocean and atop the highest peaks, craft miracle materials, light up the night, lasso the sun's energy, and build a self-reflective brain. . . . Living things have done everything we set out to do, without guzzling fossil fuel, polluting the planet, or mortgaging their future. What better models could there be?"

Some of these biomimetic applications will have medical ramifications. The unique lens structure of lobster eyes, for example, has inspired the design of a new type of telescope. This, in turn, is leading to the development of a much speedier microprocessor that, if successful, could amplify the speed of robotic testing of new drugs in the laboratory. Termite nests in arid regions are being studied because of an ingenious design that allows maximum circulation of air entering from the outside, keeping the nest cool. These nests could conceivably lead us to more efficient air-conditioning, including a system that does not harbor the Legionnaires' disease–causing bacteria that inhabit current units. The adhesives that barnacles manufacture so they can adhere to wood pilings underwater may not only teach us how to produce better paints for ships, but also enlighten us on how to synthesize new dental adhesives. And the incredibly lightweight yet strong and efficient limbs of insects and other arthropods are helping us improve the designs of everything from industrial cranes to artificial limbs.

Still, as we have seen, the study and protection of nature offers enormous direct medical benefits as well. The investigation of marine organisms, for example, has been fundamental to our understanding of the human body and how to protect it from disease. The study of both cone snail poisons and the giant nerve cells of the squid have increased our comprehension of the form and function of our nervous systems by elucidating how nerve cells communicate with each other. The lowly sea squirt, which, according to Dr. Eric Chivian of Harvard Medical School, is the only species (in addition to our own) that forms stones in its kidneylike organs, has illuminated how kidney stones form in humans. The horseshoe crab has helped us understand how eyes actually see, and studies of the sea urchin have taught us much of what we know about human development.

Well-known species may contribute to the way we heal, even if the creature is not providing us with a therapeutic compound. For example, in the winter, bears may hibernate for almost five months, during which they do not lose bone mass: the only vertebrate capable of this physiological feat. Chivian has pointed out that humans rendered immobile for this length of time—from astronauts to victims of paralysis—can lose over one-quarter of their bone mass. Deciphering how bears survive their hibernation with strong bones might help us treat and prevent osteoporosis, which affects twenty-five million Americans, causes fifty thousand deaths annually, and is estimated to cost the U.S. economy ten billion dollars per year. And how are bears able to sleep for so long without getting bedsores, while immobile humans develop such sores after only a few days? How do these hibernating creatures go for months without urinating, whereas a human being would develop uremic blood poisoning within a matter of days? Solving this enigma might help develop treatments for kidney failure, which costs the United States seven billion dollars per year.

In the recent past, some who have attempted to define what distinguishes us from other members of the animal kingdom have said that we are a species that employs medicine to treat its illnesses, but, as sometimes happens in science, "facts" and "definitions" of the past are being disproved. Perhaps it would be more accurate to define us as a species that travels the world in search of new medicines to treat its illnesses. Some of the earliest written accounts of human activity report trekking to faraway lands in search of healing substances. The most remarkable figure in the early history of what has become known as "bioprospecting" is Queen Hatchepsut of ancient Egypt. Married to her half-brother Thutmose II, she and her husband ascended to the throne in about 1512 B.C. When the king died several years later, Hatchepsut became regent for the young Thutmose III. Believing she was destined for greater things, she then had herself crowned as pharaoh and donned full pharaonic regalia (including a false beard!). In 1495 B.C., determined to expand commercial ties with the outside world, she dispatched an expedition south to the Land of Punt (Somalia) under the leadership of Prince Nehasi. Although the Egyptians returned home with gold, ivory, ebony, baboons, and dogs, the most valuable quarry they sought—and found—was myrrh, the resin of a rare tree. The thirty-one trees brought back by the expedition were planted in the temple of Amon at Thebes. This achievement was immortalized in wall carvings at the spectacular funerary temple Hatchepsut commissioned at Dayr al-Bahri.

Myrrh was prized so highly because it served as the principal antibiotic of the ancient world (note that, in strict medical terminology, the term *antibiotic* refers only to a substance produced by fungi; I am following the colloquial custom of using the term for a substance that kills bacteria). Though long regarded by some historians as merely a fragrance, myrrh was used by healers in ancient Egypt, Greece, Rome, and Persia to dress wounds. In fact, it is the most commonly mentioned wound medicine in Hippocrates' writings. Experiments in London have proven that myrrh (and the closely related frankincense) is antifungal, anti-inflammatory, and relieves the discomfort caused by both asthma and lung infections. Research in Italy demonstrated that myrrh has pain-relieving properties as well, which is probably why it was administered to Jesus prior to his crucifixion. Studies in India showed that species closely related to myrrh lower serum cholesterol levels and prevent heart disease and arteriosclerosis. When tested in the laboratory by physician Guido Majno and his colleagues in the early 1970s, myrrh proved to be extremely effective at killing *Staphylococcus*, a typical wound bacteria. Frankincense, the resin of a tree closely related to myrrh, has similar properties. So the Gift of the Magi (gold, frankincense, and myrrh) given to Jesus, Joseph, and Mary two thousand years ago was not merely some precious metal and two room deodorizers to make the barn smell better. It was the gift of life itself—the most essential medicine of the ancient world.

We in the Western world tend to think of ancient civilizations' medical practices as primitive, which many of them were. Yet the ancients' use of natural compounds was sometimes sophisticated, and our rejection of everything associated with these practices is sometimes shortsighted. The failure to value or at least investigate bacteria-killing agents like myrrh may have greatly delayed the "antibiotic revolution" for many years and cost many lives in the process. As Majno pointed out in his investigation, the Egyptians were just learning to write in 3000 B.C., but were importing massive amounts of myrrh a few hundred years later (by 2500 B.C., King Sahure had purchased eighty thousand "measures" of the aromatic substance). Over a century after Hatchepsut's death, Amenophis IV (who had already been the recipient of two boxes of myrrh as a wedding present) received a letter from a lieutenant in Palestine, which concluded:

And let the King, my Lord, send troops to his servants, and let the King, my Lord, send myrrh for medicine.

Industrialized countries still rely on nature for medicine to a much higher degree than almost anyone realizes. Almost half of all the best-selling pharmaceuticals in the early 1990s were natural products or their derivatives. A recent study of the 150 major pharmaceuticals showed that 100 percent of the drugs employed for dermatological, gynecological, or hematological purposes; 76 percent of those used for allergy, pulmonary, and respiratory purposes; 76 percent used to treat infectious diseases; and 75 percent employed for general medicine and analgesic purposes are derived from or based on natural products. Even more striking, these figures are based on "mainstream" medicines. Yet a recent Harvard Medical School study found that Americans are spending ten billion dollars per year on "alternative" or "complementary" therapies (meaning *in addition to* the medicines listed above)—many of which rely on natural products like herbs. Increased reliance on natural products is clearly on the upswing, whether it be complementary therapies like herbalism or mainstream wonder drugs from major pharmaceutical companies.

Most physicians know that aspirin is somehow related to willow bark, and many anesthesiologists are aware that general anesthesia is somehow tied to Amazonian curare vines. But I've never met a virologist who understood the connection between coral reefs and the AIDS cocktail (as we will see in Chapter 7). And, generally, most health-care practitioners are simply unaware of how dependent we are on nature for our medicines.

Nonetheless, we have to be careful to avoid the oversimplification that nature has *all* the answers to our medical problems (a surprisingly common sentiment among a certain segment of our population). Yet none other than Bill Gates (not a noted nature lover!) recently said that the growth industries of the future were information technology (presumably he meant Microsoft) and biotechnology. As we will see, it is biotechnology—the manipulation of plants and animals to produce goods useful to our own species—that is a primary force driving this search for medicines in nature. This marriage of Mother Nature's bounty to human laboratory wizardry was already worth over two billion dollars in the early 1990s and is expected to be in the tens of billions shortly after the turn of the century.

In 1968, Gordon Moore of the Intel Corporation made a remarkably prescient prediction now known as Moore's law: every eighteen months, the power of computers would double while the price of microchips would halve. The revolution that has swept the computer industry is producing a similar effect in the pharmaceutical sector. New lab techniques and instruments allow us to find new and useful compounds that occur in mind-bendingly tiny amounts. Just a few decades ago, chemists would need pounds and pounds of a plant species to isolate a new chemical compound; now they do it with a few twigs. Robochemistry—the automation and refinement of much of the drudge work of laboratory analysis—is speeding up aspects of drug development by as much as 50 percent and, in some instances, reducing costs by up to 90 percent. Given the advances in analytical techniques and the robotic automation of many mindless (but time-consuming) repetitive tasks, a cutting-edge laboratory can test over ten thousand compounds in a week. Dr. Gordon Cragg of the National Cancer Institute notes that his office screened over thirty thousand plant samples for their anti-cancer potential between the years 1958 and 1980. Now they are able to test that many samples in a year. In some cases, a single scientist can now analyze in a month what she or he would have been able to examine in an entire career just a few decades back.

Combinatorial chemistry—whereby scientists take a promising molecule and modify it to increase potency and/or reduce toxicity—adds to the likelihood that a new compound will, in one form or another, make it to market. Aspirin, the world's most commonly consumed medicine, is the best example. In 1897, the German chemist Felix Hoffman was working with salicylic acid, a plant-derived compound known to relieve pain but also to cause upset stomach. By adding some carbon and hydrogen he changed the compound into acetylsalicylic acid, which offered the same therapeutic benefits but without the unpleasant side effect.

While today's scientists can synthesize new molecules from scratch at a pace unimaginable to Hoffman, they know that Mother Nature has been creating interesting chemicals for 3.5 billion years. Why not also test those? Why not use these compounds as building blocks to be manipulated into more effective and/or less unpleasant forms than the original chemical, much as Hoffman did? The pharmaceutical industry is increasingly attuned to bizarre and promising compounds produced by nature's most creative creatures. Time and again, we discover that plants and animals produce compounds that chemists would never devise in their wildest dreams (and chemists *do* dream of chemicals in their wildest dreams). "There is simply no way that chemists would have invented the anticancer compound taxol [from the yew tree] from scratch. It is too fiendishly complex a chemical structure," said Dr. Cragg. Pharmacologist Dr. Ryan Huxtable of the University of Arizona Medical School echoed these sentiments in describing a useful chemical extracted from Hawaiian blue-green algae. "The structural variation," he said, "is one beyond the imagination of a synthetic organic chemist uncued by nature."

A significant sector of the pharmaceutical industry in the near future will marry the healing potions of the medicine man with the microchip. Contrary to what many believe, for the foreseeable future, *the value of nature as a source of novel compounds with therapeutic applications increases (rather than diminishes) as technology advances.*

More mundane than the microchip revolution, but perhaps equally important to developing new drugs from nature, is simply better transportation. When the great Harvard ethnobotanist Richard Evans Schultes tested Amazonian vision vines collected by the British explorer Richard Spruce over a hundred years earlier, he found that the stems of this woody climber were as hallucinogenic as they were the day they were harvested. The chemicals that cause the hallucinations were alkaloids, a type of chemical that often does not degrade over time. However, with my machete I can slash healing trees in the Amazon that will exude a yellow sap that will turn orange and then dark red, indicating that the chemical composition is changing as the exudate drips down the bark. No wonder so many plants that were dried, sent off to the lab, and arrived six months later did not exhibit the therapeutic effects claimed by the local peoples who knew them best! Now, with better transportation and actual labs in the rain forest, we can analyze potentially useful plants and animals much more quickly and easily.

We face many well-known diseases that we still cannot cure. We can *cure* a few types of cancers, but not many. We can successfully *treat* many kinds of cancers. We suffer many different viral infections, but our medicines only cure a few. For many illnesses, from pancreatic cancers to the common cold, we need new and effective remedies. According to Dr. Rob McCaleb—a respected authority on medicinal plants—well-researched plant medicines commonly used in western Europe reduce the risk of the four major natural causes of death in the United States: cancer, heart ailments, liver disease, and respiratory disease.

Holistic physician Dr. Karriem Ali recently noted,

> You could say that *all* so-called chronic and incurable diseases
> are the ailments that Western medicine is not proficient at
> curing, otherwise they would be neither "chronic" nor "incur-
> able." Examples include autoimmune disorders, toxic accu-
> mulations (e.g. asbestos), arthritis, arthralgias (e.g. bursitis)
> and related chronic inflammatory disorders; chronic pain (e.g.
> low back pain, migraines, phantom limb pain, sciatica); birth
> defects and genetic disorders; neurological disorders (e.g.
> Alzheimer's, Parkinson's); and viral disorders (herpes, etc.); to
> name but a few.

Probably the most frightening development in medicine is the
rise of drug-resistant diseases. This unforeseen occurrence is forcing us to look everywhere for new cures for the ailments once considered easily vanquished. Age-old scourges like tuberculosis and
malaria are back, threatening to kill us all.

The greatest and most immediate threat to our species lurks
not in the rain forest, but here at home, in every hospital, in every
neighborhood. In the fifty years since we began using commercial
antibiotics, we have been strikingly successful at eliminating the
bacteria that cause many infectious diseases. The bad news is that
some survivors have mutated into killer varieties that are impervious to antibiotics in current use. What this means is that, at some
point in the future, anytime you scrape your knee, cut yourself
shaving, or have an operation, you may be attacked by microbes
that we cannot kill. Scientists are going back to nature (where we
found the first antibiotics) to find new cures.

Another specter looming on the horizon is that of "new" diseases like AIDS or the Ebola virus. In reality, these diseases are
probably ancient, but they are coming into increased contact with
our species as we make inroads into once remote locales. Their
lethality and incurability have baffled infectious-disease experts.
Why are these diseases so frightening? Consider this description of
an Ebola victim from Richard Preston's *The Hot Zone:*

His blood is clotting-up, his bloodstream is throwing clots, and the clots are lodging everywhere. His liver, kidneys, lungs, hands, feet and head are being jammed with blood clots. In effect, he is having a stroke through his whole body. Clots are accumulating in his intestinal muscles, cutting off blood supply to his intestines. The intestinal muscles are beginning to die, and the intestines are starting to go slack. He doesn't seem to be fully aware of pain any longer because the blood clots lodged in his brain are cutting off blood flow. His personality is being wiped away by brain damage.

Lest you think this is the worst of it, you should know that it takes him another two pages to die.

Of course, the arrival of novel diseases and even plagues is nothing new: almost two thousand years ago, Pliny wrote, "New diseases, unknown in past years, have come to Italy and Europe." But a major difference is that years ago lethal diseases might spring up and kill everyone in the immediate vicinity before they could be transmitted to the world at large. In this age, however, jet travel can carry an infected person to the capital cities of most countries in less than twenty-four hours.

From a biological perspective, a major contributing factor to the spread of disease is what has been called "the human meat market theory." If you are a parasite, it makes perfect sense to focus your efforts on a common species. (Are you going to bother with pandas, a dwindling species comprised of only several hundred individuals, or with humans, so numerous and widespread?) The number of humans alive today is greater than the total of all people who ever lived in the past—and the rate of population growth continues to climb. According to Eric Chivian, there are one hundred times more people on earth than any land animal of comparable size that ever lived. More people means more likelihood of new diseases—some as yet unseen and/or unevolved—preying upon us.

Perhaps the most crucial factor driving the search for new medicines from nature is the increasing realization of the incredible diversity (and medical potential) that Mother Nature harbors. Field

research by a Smithsonian biologist in the jungles of Peru just ten
years ago led to the startling conclusion that we had underesti-
mated the number of life forms on the planet by *90 percent*! Needless to say, none of these unknown species have been analyzed to
see what potential benefit they may offer our own species. And
though all of the world's rain forests have been charted by satellites
and/or aerial photography, we still know relatively little about
what is happening beneath the great green canopy. When the late
Dr. Al Gentry, the greatest tropical field biologist of the twentieth
century, explored the forests of La Planada in southwest Colombia
in 1985, he collected seventeen species of wild philodendrons—sixteen of which were new to science. Almost every new major expedition in search of plants or insects returns from the rain forest
with new species. And even primates, one of the most conspicuous,
best-known, and least diverse groups (compared to insects, for example) have surprised us: Dutch primatologist Dr. Marc van Roosmalen has discovered over ten new species in Brazil alone.

Large mammals tend to be among the most conspicuous resi-
dents of an ecosystem: mere mention of the Arctic evokes visions of
seals and polar bears, while references to the savannas of East
Africa conjure up visions of elephants and lions. How many people
can name a shrub or a fungus that grows in either of these two
places? Yet we are still finding new species of large mammals. In the
forests of Indochina, scientists have encountered new species of
both deer and ox in the past ten years.

Still, the most prevalent and potentially useful species are not
going to be new bears and monkeys, but new plants, new invertebrates, and new microorganisms. Although large attractive species
like the rhino and the elephant—the so-called charismatic mega-
vertebrates—are the ones that catch the public eye, smaller, less
conspicuous, often less attractive species harbor the greatest pharmacological potential. Ryan Huxtable notes that species that are
small, immobile, sedentary, or slow-moving are more likely to live
by their chemical wits in terms of hunting (e.g., cone snails, sea
anemones) or defending themselves (e.g., plants) and are thus more
likely to yield interesting chemicals with medical potential than are

large mammals that are much more reliant on physical strength, sharp teeth, and speed. "Despite the claimed virtues of tiger penis and rhino horn, microorganisms have contributed more than mammals to the pharmacological happiness of mankind," he wrote.

In what has been called the "biological discovery of the decade," Danish scientists Dr. Peter Funch and Dr. Reinhardt Kristensen found an extraordinarily bizarre creature living on the mouthparts of the Norwegian lobster. Christened *Symbion pandora*, this organism is less than one-twentieth of an inch long—about the size of the period at the end of this sentence. After attaching itself to the lobster by means of a suction cup–like body part, it feeds by sweeping the lobster's leftovers into its mouth with a whirling ring that somewhat resembles a tiny vacuum cleaner. Its sex life is unlike anything ever seen before—sometimes larvae just grow out of the parent's posterior(!), while other times it grows a larva in its stomach or reproduces sexually. In one asexual stage, the creature produces what is called a dwarf male, which consists solely of a brain and reproductive organs (not to be confused with adult males of our own species). *Symbion* is so different from anything else on the planet that it has been placed in its own phylum. To get a better appreciation for the uniqueness of *Symbion*, consider that humans, goldfish, and brontosaurus are all classified as part of the same phylum: Chordata (vertebrates). The closest living relatives of *Symbion* are thought to be the bryozoans, also known as moss animals. These microscopic creatures form tiny colonies and attach themselves to rocks or vegetation in both salt and fresh water. One species of moss animal, known as *Bugula*, has been found to harbor anticancer compounds, and the National Cancer Institute is currently investigating them.

One of the most striking aspects of the discovery of *Symbion* is that such a weird creature was not found in the jungles of the Congo, or the depths of the ocean, or the peak of Mount Everest, but under our noses (or, under the lobster's nose, or, where the lobster's nose would be if it had one). *Symbion* was found on a well-studied, often-eaten species of lobster that lives in the ocean in the busy shipping lanes between Denmark and Sweden!

A single simple organism can exert profound changes on major aspects of both our science and our business. Consider that many industrial processes take place under conditions of high temperature and high pressure, conditions inimical to most life forms. There may be creatures that can prove useful in these industrial processes. To find them, a scientist may have to turn detective, investigating odd corners of the planet seemingly inhospitable to life. In the Great Fountain thermal pools of Yellowstone's Lower Geyser Basin, biologist Thomas Brock found one such species of microorganism in 1967. Named *Thermus aquaticus*, this tiny creature contains a DNA-copying enzyme that remains stable at high temperatures, and it has revolutionized genetic research. *T. aquaticus* is the basis of the polymerase chain reaction (PCR), which takes tiny bits of DNA and copies them in large numbers. PCR gives researchers the ability to take a tiny sample of DNA (a hair from a crime scene or a bone from an Egyptian mummy or a cell from a woolly mammoth) and produce enough for scientists to analyze. As a result, PCR is used in research labs and doctors' offices around the world and therefore is a multimillion-dollar-a-year industry.

PCR has already become an indispensable tool in diagnostic medicine. In the not-too-distant past, the doctor would swab your throat, touch the swab to a petri dish, and then wait for the microorganism to reproduce itself, a process that could take weeks. In contrast to this method—which often allowed the disease to progress before the diagnosis could be made—PCR functions as a molecular copying machine, churning out billions of duplicates of the offending microbe that can be identified and treated much more quickly and effectively. PCR is playing a vital role in the Human Genome Project, which is creating a complete map of our genes, thus offering hope for the prevention and treatment of many genetic disorders and other maladies.

Knowing that we can find a new phylum like *Symbion* in an accessible and well-known part of the ocean, and a new species like *Thermus aquaticus* in a Yellowstone hot spring, imagine what awaits us in the more remote corners of our planet!

.   .   .

In the age of the ubiquitous Internet, atlases on CD-ROMs, satellites in geosynchronous orbit, and handheld Global Positioning Systems, it sometimes feels that everything has been mapped and little or nothing remains to be explored or discovered. Yet this is clearly not the case. Even the course of certain rivers is poorly known. The major aerial radar mapping project in the Amazon in the early eighties revealed the presence of a tributary that had never appeared on a map. The noted Amazonian explorer John Hemming, now director of the Royal Geographic Society, has recently stated that current atlases contain "gross errors" in their depiction of certain Amazonian rivers. One night over drinks in Bogotá, I was poring over a map of the Amazon with the ethnobotanist Richard Evans Schultes, who had personally charted the course of a major river in Colombia, the least explored corner of South America. Schultes traced the course of a river on the map in front of us and smiled. "If the river runs as it is pictured here, then we should alert the media—we have found a body of water that flows up one side of a mountain and down the other!"

Among Schultes' many exploits was scaling the heights of several *tepuis*, the so-called Lost World sandstone mountains that rise out of the forests of the northern Amazon from Colombia to Suriname. On the summits of these peculiar peaks he found many species of plants new to science. Expeditions to these and to other *tepuis* in the ensuing years have discovered novel species of plants, birds, frogs, and insects. Yet not one of these Lost World mountains has been completely inventoried to catalog every life form—and several in the most inaccessible jungles of southeastern Colombia and southern Venezuela have yet to be climbed.

Although most of the world's other mountains have been scaled, many have not. One range in Tibet, which is both longer and taller than the Alps, has hardly been visited by outsiders both because of its remoteness and because of the Chinese government's desire to keep outsiders away from this contested corner of its empire. Entire ranges in Antarctica have never been climbed. A recent survey concluded that, of the more than four hundred peaks between seven thousand and eight thousand meters, more than 25 percent remain unscaled.

And even mountains that have been climbed still hold mysteries: once a mountain has been scaled, people tend to follow the same trail to the top. Few of the world's tallest mountains—Everest, K2, Kachenjunga—have been climbed from all sides. Needless to say, many that have been ascended still have not been studied for what species they harbor. The nineteenth-century Prussian explorer Alexander von Humboldt climbed almost to the top of the Ecuadorian volcano Chimborazo, then believed to be the tallest mountain in the world. In the course of the ascent, he noticed how the ecosystems formed bands around the volcano, with tropical animals, vegetation, and climate at the base gradually giving way to temperate systems at middle elevations, and arctic conditions near the summit even though the mountain stood near the equator; in other words, different parts of a mountain may harbor radically different species. Thus, even if all the known species of fungi and lichens on Mount Everest had been collected and studied for their therapeutic potential (which they have not), new species still await discovery on the unscaled slopes.

But more promising, more interesting, more bizarre than finding new species on mountain faces is discovering new worlds on planet earth. When I took my first science classes at Andrew H. Wilson Public School in New Orleans in the early 1960s, I was taught that solar energy was the basic building block of all life on earth. Plants would absorb this energy and convert it, via chlorophyll and photosynthesis, into carbohydrates, which would then be eaten by other creatures in the food chain. All life, I was told, was dependent on the sun's energy.

We now know this to be untrue. Investigations of the ocean's floor have found a world all but unconnected to sunlight. Scientists long believed that the seafloor was a biological desert: since no light penetrated to the bottom, little could survive or thrive there. The colossal water pressure alone—as much as three hundred times that found above the surface, enough to flatten a human being in a matter of seconds—would make life all but impossible. The few species that managed to eke out an existence in this barren wasteland were thought to do so by eating the carcasses of dead fish and other marine organisms that sunk from near the surface. Species diversity in the ocean deep was estimated to be a couple of hundred thousand.

Technological advances of the past quarter century have made it possible to study these formerly off-limits areas with small submarines built to withstand the crushing pressure. What we have found are new worlds, unlike anything ever envisioned outside the realm of science fiction. Marine biologists visiting these twilight worlds have found entire ecosystems thriving, based on energy released by the breakdown of toxic chemicals spewing out of the ocean floor from what are called hydrothermal vents. Stranger still are the so-called hyperthermophiles—bacteria living in or near these vents that *thrive in boiling water*. Industries are launching exploratory expeditions into these areas, believing that these microbes may provide the means to clean up toxic wastes since so many of them flourish on a diet of toxic chemicals. Other companies are investigating these creatures as the sources of new catalysts (like the species from Yellowstone, although these oceanic creatures thrive in water that is much hotter) and as the source of new medicines.

The sea is, in fact, the only place on our planet that compares to the rain forest in terms of its biological diversity and our ignorance of it. More than 70 percent of our planet is covered by water—and we are just beginning to harvest the pharmacy of the deep. At more than thirty thousand feet in depth, the Marianas Trench in the Pacific is deeper than Everest is high. Only two teams of researchers have even briefly visited these depths, fewer people than have stood on the surface of the moon.

The sheer number of newly discovered oceanic species boggles the mind. According to Dr. John Lambshead of the Natural History Museum in London, species diversity in the ocean is higher than that of all terrestrial ecosystems added together. He estimates that the ocean is home to approximately one hundred million species.

As if finding a new ocean world, totally unreliant on the energy of the sun, was not strange enough, explorers have now found an eerily parallel system here on land (or slightly under it). In the mid-1980s, the Romanian dictator Nicolae Ceauşescu ordered a nuclear reactor built in a region near the Black Sea between the Danube and the Casimcea Valley. While carrying out preliminary excavations in a cornfield to learn more about local soil conditions and suitability for the reactor's construction, the engineers broke into an uncharted underground cavern. They immediately noted the sickening stench of escaping hydrogen sulfide gas, the characteristic smell of rotting eggs. Exploration of the 160-foot-deep cavern revealed a world unlike any ever seen. The cave—christened "Movile"—was open to the outside world until approximately five million years ago, when the entrances were sealed by geological changes. Locked inside what has been called a limestone safe-deposit box was a cross-section of ancient creatures that had evolved into a range of new species. Most of the creatures had lost both their ability to see and their pigmentation (of what use are eyes or camouflage where there is zero light?). There had been a concomitant enlargement of antennae and/or antennae-like structures to allow the organisms to navigate in total darkness. Studies in Movile Cave have found forty-seven new species of spiders, leeches, and microbes.

Even more intriguing is that these creatures exist and thrive without energy input from the sun. Like the beasts that flourish around the hydrothermal vents that crease the ocean floor, these creatures have created their own ecosystem based on a toxic substance—in this particular case, hydrogen sulfide. The immediate scientific payoff is unlikely to be a new medicine. Romanian scientists and their colleagues are studying Movile to learn more about basic biology: How do species exist without photosynthesis? How do they adapt to conditions of total darkness? How fast does evolution take place? One day, perhaps, the bacteria from the cave will be used to turn poisonous industrial by-products into harmless recyclable materials. Or maybe, one day, the leeches in the cave will provide us with a new anticoagulant such as we are now obtaining from better-known species of bloodsuckers.

Despite the fact that people once lived in caves, most caverns are understudied and underexploited ecosystems from a bioprospecting perspective. Our sheer ignorance of their contents is staggering. Exploration of the deepest and most extensive cave system in the world, located in the land of the magic-mushroom cults in southern Mexico, is in the initial stages. More than 60 percent of the caves in England and 90 percent of those in Ireland have been incompletely explored—imagine the situation in tropical areas! Movile Cave, in particular, provides one more vivid example of how we have yet to learn about the world around us.

Though the phrase *the Age of Discovery* tends to conjure up images of Columbus and Magellan, more information about new species and their potential utility for humankind will be discovered in the next half century than has been found in the past five thousand years. With the estimates of global species diversity being revised from 3 million to as high as 125 million, the "supply" of potential medicines is much higher than we ever thought possible.

It is, however, a resource at risk. Relentless population growth and environmental destruction is wreaking ever greater havoc on the natural resources that offer so much promise. Accelerated rates of destruction and extinction are *not* figments of environmentalists' imagination. The golden toad, symbol of conservation in Costa Rica (the most environmentally minded country in tropical America), went extinct in the late 1980s. The elephant bird, the dodo, the Carolina parakeet—all disappeared within historical times. And many lesser-known and less-publicized species are also in trouble. Two species of medicinal mushrooms employed for healing purposes by Mazatec Indian shamans in southern Mexico have gone extinct in the past half century.

And tribes themselves continue to disappear. This is just as great a tragedy, because almost every plant or plant derivative employed for medicinal purposes by Western society was investigated scientifically after being observed in use by "primitive" cultures.

Everything from codeine for pain to quinine for malaria to podo-
phyllotoxin for cancer is based on plants discovered by ancient
healers. Over ninety tribes have gone extinct in Brazil since the
turn of the century—and virtually none of their medicinal plant
lore was recorded before they disappeared. Other tribes stand on
the brink of extinction. The Okomoyanas of Suriname have been
reduced to one ancient individual. Still other groups may continue
to exist but are losing (or already have lost) the traditions that
made them distinct as a culture. For example, the Pataxos Indians of
Brazil have been reduced to a small number of individuals, but few
(if any) still speak Pataxos. Language alone represents an excellent
barometer of "cultural integrity," and some linguists estimate that
twenty languages go extinct each year. As many as 25 percent of
the world's six thousand languages are considered highly endangered, and half of these may disappear within the next century.
Species (and the tribes that best know how to utilize them) are disappearing faster than we can count them, much less study them.
How ironic that, just as we develop the tools for unlocking some of
nature's secrets—secrets that have the potential to cure our ills,
feed the hungry, and create employment—we are destroying the
resources we are increasingly capable of utilizing.

Perhaps the most underappreciated yet eloquent spokesman on
this topic is the classics scholar Dr. John Riddle, professor of history
at North Carolina State. With his cherubic smile, gentle demeanor,
and Julius Caesar haircut, Riddle would not look out of place if he
were dressed in a toga and delivering an oration to his fellow sena-
tors in ancient Rome. Riddle is a walking encyclopedia on the medicines of the ancient world, and laces his lectures on the topic with
a razor-sharp wit. I once sat on a panel with him at a Smithsonian
conference on medicinal plants. An audience member asked us to
define the difference between a food and a drug, which generated
considerable discussion but no consensus. When it was Riddle's
turn to address this seemingly intractable issue, he paused, smiled
sweetly, and then said, "A drug is that which acts on the body while
a food is that which a body acts on." He waited while we all con-

gratulated him on his insight before noting, "Galen said that eighteen hundred years ago."

Riddle's most fascinating finding is that the ancient Greeks and Romans had a safe and widely used female contraceptive based on a species of wild fennel native to North Africa. Know as siliphion to the Greeks and silphium to the Romans, it quickly became the economic staple of the Greek city-state of Cyrene, which encompassed most of the plant's natural distribution. Silphium was well known to the ancient world, mentioned in the writings of Pliny, Hippocrates, Dioscorides, and even in a play by Aristophanes. So highly prized was the plant that it was worth more than its weight in silver and was portrayed on Cyrenian coins. Riddle has reported that experiments on lab rats with common fennel did indeed demonstrate contraceptive activity.

Unfortunately, they were unable to test the efficacy of silphium itself. Due to the insatiable demand for the plant in ancient Greece and Rome, silphium went extinct about fifteen hundred years ago.

Chapter Three

THE FUNGUS
AMONG US

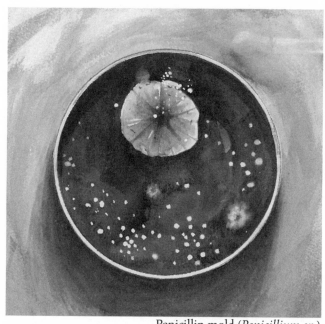

Penicillin mold (*Penicillium sp.*)

Out of the earth shall come thy salvation.
—Dr. Selman Waksman, 1944

Though merely a cousin of the lowly toadstool, the *Cordyceps* fungus lives a life that could hardly be imagined by even the most creative science-fiction writer. *Cordyceps* lies quiescent on the forest floor, waiting for its unsuspecting insect prey to pass. When a bug wanders by, the fungus attaches itself to the insect exoskeleton. It then secretes a chemical that burns a hole in the insect's body armor. Next, *Cordyceps* inserts itself into the insect body and proceeds to devour all of the host's nonvital organs, all the while preventing the insect from dying of infection by secreting an antibiotic and a fungicide (as well as an insecticide to deter other insect predators). Once the nonvital organs are consumed, the fungus eats part of the insect brain, causing the insect to ascend to the top of a tall tree in the forest. At this point, *Cordyceps* devours the rest of the bug's brain, thereby killing the insect and causing its body to split open. At that point, the fungus can release its spores a hundred feet above the forest floor.

Ironically, scientists usually refer to fungi as "lower organisms."

Mushrooms and other fungi play an enormous role in modern medicine. Five of the world's top thirty drugs are derived from fungi, penicillin being the most notable. Fungi remain one of the least studied and most promising groups of therapeutic organisms; *Cordyceps* is a case in point. Chagas' disease is a leading cause of death in some of the drier regions of South America (Charles Darwin may have died of complications resulting from contracting Chagas' in Brazil during the voyage of the *Beagle*). The disease is caused by a microorganism transmitted by the bite of the aptly named assassin beetle, which thrives in thatch huts. Chagas' is almost always fatal (although it can take decades after the initial infection); some of the Indian villages I have visited in the deserts of northern Argentina suffer up to 100 percent incidence of this disease.

Scientists are studying a species of *Cordyceps* that will invade and destroy the assassin bugs in a suitably gruesome fashion. But the medical applications, both real and potential, go further than disease prevention: Chinese Olympic runners recently set new world records in several events (the 10,000-meter event record was beaten by an extraordinary 42 seconds). The athletes attributed their record-breaking performance to a special diet, which included *Cordyceps*!

Although most Western practitioners have never heard of this unusual fungus, several Asian species are highly valued in China. The ancient Chinese employed *Cordyceps* for everything from impotence to backache; in the early 1700s, it was worth more than four times its weight in silver. Recent clinical studies have confirmed its effectiveness for treating loss of sexual drive among the elderly—making *Cordyceps* a fungal version of Viagra.

And new uses keep turning up. In 1996, Kathie Hodge, then a Cornell graduate student in mycology, was studying a Scandinavian fungus heretofore known by the jaw-breaking name *Tolypocladium inflatum*. This species is the source of the immunosuppressant drug cyclosporin, which is administered to transplant patients to prevent them from rejecting the new organs. The annual retail value of this drug is well over one hundred million dollars. As part of her teaching duties, Hodge led a group of students from her Introduction to Fungi class on a collecting field trip in a forest near the campus in upstate New York. In addition to the usual mushrooms, Hodge made an intriguing find: a dead beetle grub with a fungus sprouting from behind its head. She carefully collected the beetle carcass, taking special care not to break off the little fungus, and brought it back to the lab. Gently, Hodge placed the peculiar specimen in a laboratory dish so that the fungus could grow and change, enabling her to document its entire life cycle.

Hodge was lucky: she had found the fungus in its sexual state. Biologists know little about how to induce this state, yet without viewing the fungus's entire reproductive cycle, correctly identifying it is difficult, if not impossible. Hodge managed to get her beetle fungus to grow and change into its asexual state, convincingly demonstrating what she had suspected all along: that this fungus known as *Tolypocladium* was actually a species of *Cordyceps*, best known as the source of the drug cyclosporin. Biologists are just now learning which fungi produce this lucrative drug. Meanwhile, tens of thousands of species of fungi and other microbes have yet to be examined.

And what of the species we've examined but have yet to exhaustively utilize? In the 1950s, scientists noted that patients with cardiac problems who were taking extracts of quinine bark for malaria ceased exhibiting certain heartbeat irregularities. Further research yielded a compound in the bark, now known as quinidine, effective for treating cardiac arrhythmias. This may also prove to be the case with *Cordyceps*. The Swiss pharmaceutical giant Sandoz has isolated a compound in the fungus that it is calling NIM-811. This chemical resembles cyclosporin in terms of its molecular structure but does not suppress the immune system. What it does exhibit, however, is anti-HIV activity. Like AZT (azidothymidine), a mainstay of the anti-AIDS cocktail currently in use, NIM-811 interferes with the virus's ability to replicate. However, it disrupts the virus's reproduction at a different stage in the pathogen's reproductive cycle than does AZT. According to a recent article: "As NIM 811 acts at a different replicative stage than AZT, when the two compounds are used together in infected cell cultures they have a synergistic level of inhibition."

A popular misconception of our species' relationship with medical fungi is that it began with Alexander Fleming's study of the *Penicillium* mold in 1928. This misconception was demolished in 1991 when a German couple hiking on a high alpine ridge near the Austrian-Italian border found the corpse of a man locked in the ice of the Similaun glacier. The weather that year had been peculiar— it had been a dry winter of little snow, followed by a warm summer.

A storm known as the *foehn* had swept up from North Africa, dumping tons of sand on the Alps, causing even more ice to melt than usual. As a result, glaciers had been reduced in size throughout the mountains, and the Similaun was no exception. This exposed the upper body of the "Iceman"—caught, killed, and frozen in the ice over five thousand years earlier.

Because the Iceman was trapped in an ancient snowstorm rather than buried in a ritual grave (as is the case with most of the remains—usually mere skeletons—that scientists study), he was like a fly trapped in amber, a life literally frozen in time, the most ancient and intact person ever found—or, in all likelihood, that ever will be found. Scientists have been able to glean a wealth of information about the Neolithic culture of which he was a part. From analyzing his corpse and the materials that he carried, we learned that people cut their hair and tattooed their bodies much earlier than scientists previously believed. We found that Neolithic clothing was tailored to keep out the cold in a much more sophisticated fashion than we had thought. And we discovered that our prehistoric ancestors knew infinitely more about weapons than we ever gave them credit for: the fletching (feathers) on the arrows found with the Iceman was attached in such a way as to create spin in flight, so that the arrows would be much more likely to find their mark; this indicated a solid grasp of ballistic principles. Equally impressive was the fur strap he wore around his wrist on which he had threaded birch fungi. The European research team that carried out the original analysis of the Iceman initially hypothesized that these fungi served as kindling. We now believe that this strap represents the earliest known first aid kit.

Some fungi are dry and spongy, making them effective tinder with which to start a fire. Birch fungi, however, being difficult to light, are unsuitable for kindling. Mycologists were quick to point out that this species of fungus is rich in polyporic acid C, known to kill bacteria. The Iceman and (presumably) his compatriots appear to have employed fungi for medicinal purposes fifty centuries before Alexander Fleming.

Nor is the Iceman's fungi the only indication that ancient

peoples probably knew and used these substances for healing purposes. Consider this passage from the Ebers papyrus, written in
Egypt around 166 B.C.: "But if the wound rots too much, then bind
on it spoiled barley bread."

Classics scholar John Riddle has noted that the ancient Greeks
scraped the moldy grime from the walls of their gymnasiums and
applied it to wounds, while the Aztecs fed moldy tortillas to patients suffering from infectious diseases. Thousands of years ago,
Chinese healers applied moldy soybeans to boils and other skin infections. In ancient Greece, Dioscorides prescribed fungi for a wide
variety of ailments. The French are known to have applied moldy
cheese to infections. And English milkmaids in the Middle Ages
bound moldy bread to their wounds. I myself have had earaches (of
presumably bacterial origin) cured by Amazonian shamans who
used the sap of forest fungi. And according to David Werner and
Bill Bower in their 1984 book *Learning to Promote Health:* "In
Mexico, long before the discovery of penicillin, the rural people
[campesinos] were treating women with puerperal [childbirth]
fever by giving them a tea made of the fungus from the subterranean gardens of the leafcutter ants. It is possible that this fungus
is related to penicillin."

Fungi are one of several types of microbes, along with bacteria,
algae, and protozoa. Of the four, fungi and bacteria are of primary
importance in treating sickness. Bacteria are undoubtedly the most
ancient form of life on earth, having appeared well over three billion years ago, making them about two billion years older than any
other creature. And they are probably the most numerous and diverse form of life—the number of *E. coli* bacteria in each person is
greater than the number of all the human beings who have ever
lived. Bacteria are among the tiniest forms of life—about a quarter
of a million could fit on the period at the end of this sentence. And
they are the most ubiquitous, being found from the high peaks of
the Himalayas, to the ocean floor, to deep inside the earth's crust.
(One of the deepest probes ever inserted into the earth found bacteria all the way down!) These creatures may yet prove to be the
most numerous of all life forms. In a *New York Times* op-ed piece,

the great evolutionary biologist Dr. Stephen Jay Gould wrote: "The textbooks of my youth designated our current epoch as the Age of Man. Current linguistic preferences favor an Age of Mammals. More generous people, with fewer parochial intentions, often choose to honor a truly dominant multicellular group of more than a million described species (compared with a paltry 4000 for mammals): the Age of Insects. But all these proposals represent little more than multicellular prejudice. We are now, as our planet has been for 3.5 billion years, in an Age of Bacteria."

Biologists classify bacteria as *prokaryotes,* distinctive from all other life forms (which are classified as *eukaryotes*). Prokaryotes are tiny, single-celled creatures that lack the organized, organlike structures (like a nucleus) found in all the eukaryotes. Prokaryotes are surrounded, supported, and protected by thick cell walls made of complex sugars called polysaccharides. Only bacteria have these walls. Because animals lack these cell walls, drugs that selectively attack the walls can kill bacteria *in* the animals without harming the animals. In other words, these cell walls can be thought of as the bacterial equivalent of Achilles' heel.

Microbiologists divide bacteria into two basic types based on whether they absorb a certain dye named for the Danish scientist Cristof Gram. We say that a bacterium is "gram positive" or "gram negative." Most bacteria exert no effect on human welfare, yet some play a positive role: either indirectly, by fixing nitrogen in the soil that aids plant life, or more directly by converting milk to cheese or aiding human digestion. Bacteria are also responsible for some of our deadliest ailments: bacterial pneumonia (in terms of infectious diseases, the major cause of illness and death in the United States), cholera, diphtheria, gonorrhea, leprosy, plague, scarlet fever, syphilis, tetanus, and typhoid.

And very recent research has led some scientists to postulate that *bacteria may be the cause of many chronic ailments previously attributed to other phenomena like aging, diet, or genetics.* Supposedly noninfectious diseases like Alzheimer's, atherosclerosis (hardening of the arteries), arthritis, asthma, and cancer may be caused—or partially caused—by bacteria. Stomach ulcers, long attributed to everything from stress to poor eating habits, are now attributed to infections of *Helicobacter* bacteria. If these hypotheses about the infectious origin of supposed chronic diseases prove true, bacteria are responsible for much more human misery and death than we ever dared imagine. And the medical potential of other microbes—which have already provided us with our most successful cures for infectious diseases—is even greater than we have realized.

Fungi are not the only source of antibiotics: bacteria have yielded an even richer lode. Actinomycetes, a group of soil bacteria, have produced more commercial antibiotics than any other group of organisms. Dr. Peter Raven, director of the Missouri Botanical Garden, estimates that, of the three thousand antibiotics discovered by 1974, two thousand came from actinomycetes. In one of nature's greatest ironies, tuberculosis (one of our species' most ancient and ubiquitous killers) is an actinomycete, as is the species that produces streptomycin, the first known cure for this dreaded disease.

The diversity of microbes—bacteria, fungi, algae, and protozoa—boggles the mind. These organisms, often invisible to the naked eye, nonetheless dominate the tree of life by having more branches than any other life forms. These branches, according to Bob Holmes of *New Scientist*, feature "more than a dozen groups as different from each other as humans are from pine trees." Less than 5 percent of all species have been identified by scientists, and only a small percentage of that has been extensively screened for novel compounds. There may exist over thirteen million species of fungi, yet only seventy thousand species have been studied in the laboratory, and those that have been tested were evaluated primarily for antibiotic potential. And recent research is uncovering unimagined diversity and complexity among the bacteria.

Until relatively recently, bacteria could only be described and understood by collecting them in the wild (usually from soil samples) and growing them in the laboratory, a tedious and often inefficient practice. Using much more sophisticated analysis based on DNA extraction and then replication with the polymerase chain reaction (PCR), as well as other novel techniques, scientists are reaching astonishing conclusions. Realizing that previous techniques of collecting and censusing these organisms were spectacularly inefficient and ineffective, they now recognize that microbial diversity greatly exceeds earlier estimates. In a recent article in *New Scientist,* microbiologist Dr. John Holt of Michigan State University said, "You could go out in your backyard and if you really put your mind to it, you could find a thousand new species in not much time." Experiments by Norwegian scientist Dr. Vidgis Torsvik found evidence of ten thousand different types in a gram of soil— approximately two times more species of bacteria than have ever been described by science. We not only have to revise sharply upward our estimate of the number of species on earth, but also to realize what a medical treasure trove the microbial kingdom remains despite the wonder drugs it has already provided.

Biologically, fungi are plantlike organisms that lack chlorophyll and typical plant organs like leaves, stems, and roots. Unlike plants (which manufacture their own food), fungi must feed on other organisms, which they accomplish by secreting enzymes and absorbing the nutrients. As with bacteria, they thrive almost everywhere: in air, soil, water, food, and in and on the human body. They are mostly tiny, but also include the largest organism of all time: a one-thousand-year-old, two-and-a-half-square-mile underground fungus discovered in southwest Washington State in 1992.

Like bacteria, fungi maintain something of a love-hate relationship with our species. These microorganisms cause human diseases like athlete's foot, ringworm, and histoplasmosis, and are responsible for plant diseases like chestnut blight and Dutch elm disease. Fungi affect our lives in many beneficial ways as well: they produce enzymes employed in industry; parasitize and kill harmful insects (remember *Cordyceps!*); consume and detoxify toxic chemicals; and enhance the growth of certain trees. Yeasts (which are actually microscopic fungi) play a key role in the production of beer, bread, and wine. And mushrooms and their relatives are dietary staples in many human cultures.

As we saw with the Iceman, fungi have long been used for medical purposes, and new uses are constantly being developed. In the past thirty years, cyclosporin from *Cordyceps* has produced a major immunosuppressant; coprine from the inkcap mushroom (which induces nausea when mixed with alcohol) has been given to alcoholics to dissuade them from drinking; and a patent has been taken out on the branching filaments of mucor mushrooms as a wound dressing because these structures retain moisture and promote rapid healing when applied to the affected area. A soil fungus served as the basis for Merck's blockbuster drug lovastatin (Mevacor), used to lower blood cholesterol levels. Thousands of fungi species have been evaluated almost solely for antibiotic properties, but hundreds of thousands—if not millions—remain to be tested.

The medical interest in microbes can be attributed to warfare, not between people, but among microscopic organisms. When we think of the struggle for survival among species, Tennyson's famous line about "nature red in tooth and claw" often comes to mind, but bacteria and fungi were battling each other long before nature evolved the first tooth, the first claw, or the first red blood. These microorganisms, in all likelihood, will still be warring with each other long after humans have departed from the scene. Western medicine's use of antibiotics is mostly predicated on filching the weapons that fungi have spent three billion years developing to combat other microorganisms and aiming them at microbes that attack humans.

In a world awash in antibiotics, it is difficult to comprehend how common in the recent past death due to infectious disease was. Pneumonia, still prevalent today, was not long ago considered a lethal scourge, killing one-third of the people who contracted it. Infectious diseases once caused one-half of the deaths of all children under the age of six in the United States at the turn of the century. A single cut while shaving could lead to death by blood poisoning. Simply being near someone who sneezed could prove fatal. Virtually all surgery and childbirth exposed people to the possibility of contracting lethal infections. And soldiers in mechanized wars like the Civil War or World War I more often died of infections than battle wounds. The discovery, commercialization, and widespread availability of safe and effective antibiotics revolutionized everything from surgical practice to warfare to urban living.

The great French scientist Louis Pasteur discovered that germs cause disease. This was by no means Pasteur's only contribution to science: he invented pasteurization, made commonplace the practice of vaccination, and personally developed the rabies vaccine. Pasteur noted that some forms of bacteria seemed to destroy others, but he never really put the idea into medical practice.

Dr. Joseph Lister, a Scottish contemporary of Pasteur, is best known as one of the first proponents of sterilization and disinfectants. If germs were everywhere, he reasoned, then might the surgeon be spreading disease from one person to the next? Lister convinced fellow surgeons to wash their hands and sterilize their instruments between operations. In 1844, Lister is said to have used a crude mold extract to cure the wound of a patient. And in 1871, Lister wrote about microbes that warred with one another, after noticing that some molds halted the growth of certain bacteria. In a fascinating note to his brother, Lister indicated that he was considering experimenting with a species of *Penicillium* mold as a surgical antiseptic (!), though there seems to be no written record as to whether he followed through on this brilliant idea.

As early as 1877, the British scientist Dr. John Tyndall noticed *Penicillium* molds killing bacteria in a test tube. But it was not until Sir Alexander Fleming's research on this fungus in the late 1920s that penicillin became an integral part of Western medicine. Nonetheless, the development of the mold extract into one of the most crucial curatives ever derived from natural sources was fraught with irony and serendipity.

Fleming was a field surgeon during World War I. Traumatized as they watched wounded soldiers suffer agonizing deaths from stinking infected wounds, he and his colleagues began searching for drugs to cure infections as soon as the war ended. In September of 1928, Fleming was studying a strain of staph bacteria that causes boils. After returning from a brief vacation in the country to his lab in a London hospital, he found that mold had invaded a petri dish on which he was growing his bacteria. Contamination usually causes scientists to immediately discard the petri dish and start over, but Fleming had a reputation as a patient and skilled observer. Looking carefully at the plate, he noted that the mold seemed to be advancing on the bacteria and turning the staph into a watery mush. Intrigued, Fleming photographed the petri dish on which this microtitanic battle was raging. This photograph recorded a turning point in the relationship between man and microbe.

Fleming scraped off a bit of the mold and added it to a test tube filled with a culture medium, a substance on which the mold could feed and grow. From the outset, he had trouble cultivating sufficient quantities for experimentation. He injected penicillin into healthy mice and they were unaffected, indicating that the drug was not particularly toxic. Fleming then applied penicillin to external wounds and found they healed quickly and without complication.

For a drug to be effective in the body, it has to be able to attack the invader without (ideally) causing any harm to the person. Unlike vaccines, which destroy infectious diseases by working with the body's immune system, antibiotics function by direct attack on disease-causing organisms (while a vaccine can be thought of as instructors who come in and train the troops, antibiotics can be considered hired guns brought in from outside to conduct the actual fighting). An effective method entails aiming your "smart bomb" at targets found only in bacterial cells. This is precisely how penicillin functions. Penicillin's target is the enzyme that the bacterial cell employs to help build its unique wall. Without the enzyme, the cell is unable to construct its outer wall and, without the wall, the cell eventually bursts and dies. Other antibacterials function by interfering either with cellular reproduction or the permeability of the cell membrane, thereby causing the bacteria to lose control of what can enter or leave the cell. Bacteria can no more survive without the support of their walls than could a human survive without its skeleton.

So penicillin might have seemed like an ideal drug—but Fleming's remarkable discovery went relatively unnoticed. A careful and cautious man by nature, Fleming failed to take the next step, which seems obvious in retrospect: he never injected the new drug into sick creatures to learn whether his new find could cure internal infections. He published his results in 1929, eliciting little response from the medical community.

Serendipity is a recurrent theme in the search for new medicines and, indeed, in almost all aspects of science. Not surprisingly, scientists prefer to convey the perception that every discovery begins with a simple hypothesis that, after testing, results in a logical conclusion. Some momentous discoveries are made that way, but many are not. The truly revolutionary discoveries—those that transform society and the course of civilization, as penicillin most certainly has—often result from a mixture of luck and a lightning-like strike of blinding insight that leads to something new.

Scientists' inability to re-create Fleming's petri-dish experiment for almost forty years proves that serendipity played a role. Even Fleming himself tried it again, many years later, without success. A petri dish would be left near an open window, but the same species of *Penicillium* mold failed to appear. Or the correct species of *Penicillium* would be added to a petri dish full of staph bacteria but the bacteria would not be killed. What made Fleming's breakthrough in September 1928 possible?

The answer may have been the location of Fleming's laboratory. In late 1928, mycologist C. J. La Touche was studying various molds and their relationships to allergies just two floors below Fleming's lab in St. Mary's Hospital. Perhaps his mold landed in Fleming's lab, making the growth of that particular penicillin species possible. Both an elevator shaft and a stairway, either of which could have served as the path between the Irishman's office and the Scot's petri dish, connected the two laboratories. The weather had been unseasonably cool, another factor that would have contributed to the fungi's exuberance. And we now know that penicillin works by keeping bacteria from building cell walls, meaning that it does not kill mature bacteria but keeps the less mature forms from reproducing. When subsequent experiments involving a petri dish with equal parts *Penicillium* mold and mature staph bacteria were tested, the results were more of a standoff than a victory by the "miracle mold." Without this unique juxtaposition of events, the discovery and development of events might have occurred decades later.

And warfare—this time, among members of our own species—played a role. By the winter of 1940–41, international headlines focused not on new antibiotics but on the seemingly unstoppable advance of Hitler's armies. The Germans had overrun France and occupied much of western Europe; the Soviet armies were falling back in the face of the Nazi onslaught. Hitler's generals were preparing for Operation Sea Lion, the invasion and conquest of the British Isles. The need to improve treatment of wounds on the battlefield would prove to be the decisive factor in the commercial development of the drug.

An Oxford University research team led by the Australian Dr. Howard Florey picked up where Fleming left off. Florey had first learned of penicillin from a colleague who had obtained some of the original mold from Fleming. The Australian found it difficult to grow a sufficient quantity to study in detail. Dr. Ernst Chain, a Jewish-German refugee, joined Florey's research team and urged his new boss to persist. Thus a Jew fleeing Hitler played a leading role in developing the drug that aided in the Allies' defeat of the Third Reich. Chain later admitted that he became interested in the project "not because I hoped to discover a miracle drug . . . but because I thought it had great scientific interest!"*

---

*Ironically, antibiotics did not initially come to the fore because of natural products: the first antibiotic to excite the Western scientific community was actually a novel use of the synthetic dye prontosil red, developed by the Germans. Chemist Gerald Domagk (who was forbidden to leave Germany to accept a Nobel Prize for his efforts because his pacifist inclinations enraged the Nazi hierarchy) tested this dye in mice that he had injected with the deadly strep bacteria. Ironically, the dye did not kill the bacteria in the test tube, but when the chemist gave it to the infected mice, they all survived and thrived. Later investigation reconfirmed Domagk's thesis that the dye was broken down in the body in separate components, one of which—sulphanilamide—was the effective antibiotic compound. As an additional bonus, sulphanilamide did not turn the patient bright red, unlike prontosil. This drug, developed by the Germans, was used in the late 1930s to save the lives of both Franklin Delano Roosevelt, Jr., and Winston Churchill!

Florey's team generated promising results in the lab: rodents injected with penicillin survived the injection of deadly strep bacteria. The next step entailed testing the drug on humans suffering from bacterial infections, and the results were sensational: patients who would have died without the drug were making miraculous recoveries. Demand far outstripped supply. British scientists were growing *Penicillium* molds on cookie tins and bedpans. Penicillin was so precious that it was extracted from the urine of treated patients for reuse (curiously reminiscent of a practice of peasants in Siberia, who would sometimes drink the urine of wealthy locals who had imbibed the hallucinogenic fly agaric mushroom—as is the case with penicillin, the chemicals are not destroyed in the body).

Florey and his team were convinced of the strategic importance of their find. If the Nazis succeeded in conquering England, the scientists were determined to flee to America where the results of their research might one day serve the Allied cause. Worried that the Germans would confiscate their test tubes, Florey's men prepared for this eventuality by rubbing reproductive *Penicillium* spores into their clothing. British industry, struggling for survival, had no time and less money to spend on experimental research. Florey had already received some grant monies from the Rockefeller Foundation in New York—might the Foundation be interested in increasing their support of research that might one day prove to be of paramount strategic importance to America's military forces should they enter the war?

Accompanied by lab technician Norman Heatley, the man who best knew how to grow the mold, Florey traveled to a secret airstrip where he boarded a blacked-out airplane for a flight to Lisbon, which, neutral in the war, swarmed with refugees and spies of both the Allied and the Axis powers. Once in Lisbon, the two Englishmen and their precious cargo boarded a Pan Am clipper seaplane for the twenty-four-hour flight to New York. They arrived at La Guardia's Marine Air Terminal on July 2, 1941.

Two weeks later, with the aid of the Rockefeller Foundation, they were meeting with the director of the newly established regional research laboratory of the United States Department of

Agriculture in Peoria, Illinois. Here, Heatley and his American co-horts made several revolutionary advances in the production of penicillin. Located in the heart of the Midwest, the new USDA facility was determined to find new uses for corn and corn by-products. One of the first experiments by the British-American team was to try cultivating the mold on corn-steep liquor, the stinky residue that remained from a process in which starch was extracted from corn. The mold thrived on this new foodstuff, producing over twenty times more penicillin than ever before. Heatley and his American colleagues were determined to boost yields even further. They were growing the mold on the surface of the corn-steep liquor. Could it be grown throughout the liquor (the so-called deep-fermentation method) and produce more of the precious drug?

Penicillium notatum did not thrive under these conditions. Scientists wondered if another species might do better. Dr. Kenneth Raper, the mycologist at Peoria, enlisted the assistance of the U.S. Army Transport Command and, in short order, soil samples poured in from every corner of the globe. The superlative strain proved to be a yellow species of *Penicillium*—found growing on a rotten cantaloupe in a Peoria market! *Penicillium chrysogenum* not only yielded much more penicillin than Fleming's original mold, but also thrived in deep fermentation. It has been called the grand-daddy of all penicillin products used today.

By late 1942, only about one hundred people in the United States had been treated with penicillin. Just three years later, near the end of the war, penicillin had saved millions of lives. Even its emotional contribution to the Allied cause cannot be overstated: German soldiers wounded in battle often died of the same infections that had killed their fathers and grandfathers in the trenches during the previous war. Many Allied soldiers would suffer the same wounds but, after the administration of the new mold-derived drug, would experience a Lazarus-like resurrection to fight again.

Merck Pharmaceuticals (headed by George Wilhelm Merck, of German ancestry) played a pioneering role (under a program directed by Max Tishler, a Jew who had been denied a job at DuPont because of his religion) in producing quantities of penicillin sufficient to meet the needs both on the Allied battlefront and the home front. Penicillin, used to treat the victims of the horrendous 1943 Coconut Grove nightclub fire, proved particularly effective against the staph bacteria that flourished in the damaged skin of the burn victims. So effective were the results that the U.S. government and pharmaceutical companies ratcheted up production sufficient to meet all military needs within eighteen months. (The Allies' "secret weapon" receives scant mention in many historical accounts of World War II, although Graham Greene's novel *The Third Man* focuses on the black market for the drug in postwar Europe.)

Penicillin was not the only natural product essential to the war effort. Troops suffering from malaria in much of the Pacific theater could only be cured by the bark of the *Cinchona* tree. Because Japanese forces had captured Southeast Asia's *Cinchona* plantations at the outset of the war, Smithsonian botanist Dr. Raymond Fosberg was sent to South America to find some of the original high-yielding strains of the trees. One night, in a fleabag hotel in a remote locale high in the Andes of southern Colombia, he heard a conversation in German and a knock at his door. He opened the door to find two Nazi agents who had been tracking him. His heart skipped a beat until they explained that they wished to sell him a contraband shipment of quinine, which he quickly agreed to purchase, both to help the troops in the Pacific and, he decided, himself.

Quinine was considered essential to the war effort in the Pacific; more Americans were dying from malaria than from Axis bullets. In mid-1944, the giant Japanese submarine *I-52* departed from its homeport and headed for a secret Atlantic rendezvous with a German U-boat. The assignment: trade Japan's most valuable raw materials for German weapons technology. On the night of June 23, 1944, *I-52* met up with German *U-530*. Allied cryptographers had cracked the Axis codes, however, and an American bomber sank the Japanese sub, killing everyone on board. Fifty years later, using sonar technologies developed in the search for the *Titanic*, explorer Paul Tidwell found the sub in seventeen thousand feet of water.

What had the sub been carrying when she was spotted and sunk? Gold, rubber, and three tons of quinine.

No single antibiotic ever has been (or ever will be) an effective killer of all disease-causing bacteria. From the very beginning of the antibiotic revolution, different antibiotics provided different degrees of efficacy against different types of bacteria (for example, penicillin is the drug of choice for treating throat infections caused by one sort of bacteria, while erythromycin is preferred for certain types of skin infections). The realization that other fungi produced compounds that might kill bacteria impervious to penicillin led to a worldwide search for new fungi. Chloramphenicol, originally isolated from a Venezuelan soil fungus, is active against both gram-positive and gram-negative bacteria and is particularly effective against both typhus and typhoid fever. Unlike penicillin, it kills the bacteria directly rather than prohibiting its ability to reproduce. Streptomycin, from an American soil fungus, is also active against both gram-positive and gram-negative bacteria and served as the first effective cure for tuberculosis when Selman Waksman and his colleagues at Rutgers University discovered and developed it in the early 1940s. And the mighty vancomycin, one of the most potent antibiotics ever found, comes from a fungus found in a clump of Indonesian mud.

The search for new antibiotics—and the fungi that produce them—has led to other drugs as well. The immunosuppressant cyclosporin, from the insect-killing *Cordyceps* fungus, was unearthed during a search for antibiotics, paralleling the serendipitous discovery of penicillin. H. P. Frey, a scientist employed by Sandoz, was vacationing in Norway when he collected a soil sample to be analyzed when he returned home. Little did he realize that he had stumbled across a substance that would change human-organ transplant surgery from a risky experimental procedure to a fairly routine practice!

The basic hurdle in transplant surgery: an immune system brilliantly designed to attack and kill intruders. Once a foreign organism or substance is detected in the body, the immune system is

alerted, and white blood cells sound the alarm, attacking, destroying, and sometimes devouring the intruder. If white blood cells go
into a feeding frenzy over a stray bacterium, imagine their fury
over an entire organ! But how to keep these defenders from as-
saulting a transplanted organ?

When the Swiss began testing the chemical compounds extracted from fungi in the Norwegian soil sample, they were disappointed to find that the chemicals were weak antibiotics, which
normally might not merit further research. But a computer analysis of the compounds indicated that they were a new type of chemical, unlike anything in use. When the new compound, dubbed
cyclosporin, was tested on the human immune system, it was
found to suppress the system in a unique way, by dissuading the T
cells from attacking the new tissue.

Organs and tissues as diverse as corneas, hearts, kidneys, lungs,
and spleens are now transplanted on a regular basis. Cyclosporin
continues to play an indispensable role: Barney Clark, the first
heart transplant recipient, lived only eighteen days, while 80 percent of people undergoing the same procedure now survive over a
year (and many live much, much longer). This fungal product has
already generated revenues well in excess of one billion dollars, yet
it almost was discarded because it was not a powerful antibiotic—
and few laboratories were looking for immunosuppressive agents
at the time it was discovered. In the words of pharmacologist Dr.
Ryan Huxtable: "Value is a function of need and, as it is difficult to
predict future needs, it is difficult to conclude that a species currently without value will always remain so. . . . Who 30 or 40 years
ago could have predicted the need for immunosuppressants such as
cyclosporin? Without such agents, tissue and organ transplants
would be impossible. . . . We cannot predict what new needs may
arise based on insights and discoveries yet to be made."

Though antibiotics have long been heralded as "miracle drugs,"
a fearsome threat to our species has appeared on the horizon: drug-
resistant bacteria. The popularity of books like Preston's *The Hot
Zone* and films like *Outbreak* has led to fear of killer viruses like
Ebola. Though Ebola, or the lesser-known but equally dangerous

varieties like Bolivian hemorrhagic fever, are mostly found in far-off jungles of the humid tropics, drug-resistant bacteria are common in places closer to home, like our neighborhood hospital. Diseases like bacterial pneumonia, blood poisoning, syphilis, and tuberculosis, once considered relatively easy to cure, have all developed strains resistant to some antibiotics. *Virtually every disease-causing bacterium is known to have an antibiotic-resistant strain.* According to the Centers for Disease Control and Prevention (CDC), over thirteen thousand patients in the United States were killed by drug-resistant bacterial strains in 1992 alone.

The "killer microbe" phenomenon has captured the attention of the media—warranting cover stories in both *Time* and *Newsweek*—but the danger of the situation was evident at the outset. As early as 1945, Alexander Fleming himself highlighted the danger in an interview published in the *New York Times*. True to his prediction, several scientists began finding staph bacteria resistant to penicillin in 1946, despite the fact that the medicine only became widely available five years before that. Though streptomycin, the first cure for tuberculosis, was first isolated in 1943, TB strains resistant to the drug were noted as early as 1947.

Bacteria have developed several frighteningly ingenious methods for defusing antibiotic smart bombs. A common defense is the production of substances that destroy the antibiotic before it can demolish the bacteria: some varieties of the staph bacteria produce a compound called penicillinase, which obliterates the penicillin molecule. Yet another trick is for the bacteria to change its outer membrane so that the antibiotic is unable to enter the cell. Still another tactic is for the bacteria to "vomit" the antibiotic out of its cell.

Bacteria reproduce and evolve extraordinarily quickly, making resistance almost a mathematical certainty. On average, it takes twenty years for people to produce a new generation of offspring. Each generation represents a new combination of genetic material, potentially improving their ability to survive. Bacteria, on the other hand, can reproduce in ten minutes. One bacterium can produce almost 17 million progeny in a twenty-four-hour period, or

8,160,000,000 progeny in the time it takes us to mature, mate, and produce our first child. Of the 17 million produced in a single day, *only a single bacterium* has to prove to be drug-resistant to initiate the whole chain of events.

Use of antibiotics facilitates the creation, evolution, development, and spread of the resistant strains. Once the patient has taken the drug, the drug-sensitive strains are killed off, leaving only the resistant forms to multiply and take over. Another exceedingly common phenomenon that aids and abets drug-resistant strains is the misuse of the medicine: how many of us have been instructed to take all the prescribed pills and, instead, stopped halfway through the supply because we "felt better"? This all-too-common occurrence, whereby the bacteria faces a sublethal dose, permits the bug to figure out how best to adapt to the drug. Furthermore, physicians sometimes inappropriately use the most powerful antibiotics like vancomycin when a less potent drug might have sufficed. The result is, of course, vancomycin-resistant strains, meaning that this drug—the treatment of last resort—will no longer be effective as the ultimate cure when other antibiotics don't work. Two additional culprits are patients who demand the most powerful antibiotics, even for viral diseases that cannot be cured by antibiotics, and pharmaceutical companies anxious to market their new wares to maximize returns on large research and development budgets.

Exacerbating the resistance problem is the prevalence of antibiotics in most of our meat and milk. Antibiotics not only fight infections in farm animals; they also help them grow faster. Feed manufacturers often add antibiotics directly to the grains. How many people realize that federal law permits milk to contain traces of eighty different antibiotics?

The elimination of common, well-understood, and easily treatable bacteria in hospitals opens an ecological niche for other bacteria that can prove impervious to commonly used medications. And changes in society have also contributed to the problem. International jet travel means that infectious diseases can be moved from one side of the planet to the other in twenty-four hours. The prevalence of the AIDS virus has created a huge population in which bacteria can flourish in a way not possible when confronted with a healthy immune system. Huge urban populations of both the elderly and the homeless also present a population relatively amenable to disease. And finally (and most terrifying) is another newly discovered talent of bacteria: the ability to share the gene that conveys resistance to a drug not only with its own progeny but also *with entirely unrelated microbes!* One organism may transfer a piece of DNA known as a plasmid to another bacteria, much as devotees of computer games exchange tricks and shortcuts, allowing them to beat the computer at a game they may be playing for the first time. Because of this plasmid transfer, bacteria can become resistant to drugs they have yet to face.

Meanwhile, terrifying new strains of bacteria continue to evolve. We in the industrialized world smugly tend to associate infectious diseases with poor people living in poor countries, but these maladies still claim casualties here at home. Streptococcus bacteria are best known as the cause of strep throat but can cause other diseases as well, from seemingly mild ailments like impetigo to potentially more serious ones like scarlet fever. But highly virulent new strains with lethal potential continue to appear, a threat to every human being. Multimillionaire puppeteer Jim Henson, creator of the Muppets, was struck down by one of these frightening strains in 1990. Although only fifty-three and in good health, Henson died within days of contracting the disease, which causes many of the body's organs to fail. This particular strain kills four out of five of the people it infects.

As frightening (if not more so) is yet another strain of strep bacteria. Labeled "necrotizing myositis" by physicians, it is widely known by the more bloodcurdling and accurate moniker "flesh-eating bacteria." Scientists hypothesize that this strain arises when a virus invades the bacteria and causes it to pump out toxic chemicals. The bacteria targets the connective tissue (fascia) that binds the skin and muscle tissue, a flesh layer that lacks the rich network of blood vessels that carry immune cells and antibiotics to combat infections. The bacteria and the toxins it produces cut off circulation of blood to surrounding tissues, killing them. These bacteria can eat through an inch of flesh in an hour! They attacked the charismatic Canadian separatist leader Lucien Bouchard in 1994, and doctors had to inject him with megadoses of antibiotics and amputate one of his legs to save his life. If the physicians had been less aggressive in their treatment, Bouchard would certainly have died, and the political fate of Quebec and the rest of Canada may well have been determined by microbes.

In 1969, the U.S. surgeon general announced that "it was time to close the book on infectious disease," a statement that is being widely quoted these days, but not because of its acumen. The gentleman sincerely believed that, with our armentarium of antibiotics, we had microbes on the run and should shift our emphasis to killers like cancer and heart disease. The major pharmaceutical companies agreed, diverting their research and development monies away from the search for novel antibiotics. Much of the drug development in the anti-infective field from the 1950s through 1970s focused on the so-called me-too drugs, which involve incremental improvements of medicines already on the market. Today, with bacteria evolving ever faster, the race is on to develop new drugs. The question is, then, where will the new antibiotics come from?

A major source of new antibiotics will continue to be the bacteria themselves. A relatively new antibiotic derived from bacteria is Synercid, being brought to the market by French manufacturer Rhône-Poulenc. According to Dr. Harriette Nadler, a microbiologist at Rhône-Poulenc, the development of this drug was initiated when scientists extracted a complex new compound from an Argentine soil sample in 1955. It took the company seven years to analyze and test the complex chemical because it had a different structure than other antibiotics. This new class of compounds was dubbed "streptogramins" and "pristinamycins" based on the scientific name of the bacteria from which they were extracted: *Streptomyces pristinaespiralis*. The first commercial application was an oral antibiotic introduced in France in the 1960s. Synercid, which is a parenteral (injectable) drug, was developed in the 1980s.

Synercid appears to be effective against some drug-resistant bacteria because it kills them in a peculiar manner: it bonds to a key piece of the cell that prevents the microbe from producing proteins necessary for its survival. It also interferes with the bacteria's form and function by causing a thickening of the cell wall, which later dissolves. According to Dr. Nadler, this cell-wall fragmentation proves fatal to the microbe.

Synercid has captured the attention of medical practitioners because it has proven effective against two strains of bacteria resistant to vancomycin. In the past few years, several thousand Americans suffering from infections by drug-resistant bacteria had their lives saved by Synercid. But its effectiveness is already being undercut: European farmers use Synercid-like antibiotics as a feed additive. Synercid-resistant bacteria have already developed in these animals, and it is only a matter of time before these microbes attack people. In the words of Dr. Stuart Levy of Tufts Medical School, author of *The Antibiotic Paradox,* the classic book on antibiotics and drug resistance, "Synercid is not a panacea. What it does is buy us some time. Synercid will not be able to save us over the long term."

Levy strongly believes that more judicious use of current antibiotics is essential. Other scientists are developing the means to combat the bacterial resistance directly by trying to decipher how to keep the bacteria from being able to pump the tetracycline out of the cell or being able to chop the penicillin molecule into tiny useless bits. If they succeed, then these "old" antibiotics can be given new life.

Though most scientists have looked to microbes for new sources of antibiotics, amphibians are now providing a promising lead from the animal kingdom. In the late 1980s, after operating on African clawed frogs to extract their eggs, Dr. Michael Zasloff of the National Institutes of Health made a curious observation: these amphibians seldom developed infected wounds, even when placed in water that was less than clean. How, he wondered, were they fending off infection from the microbes that surrounded them? Investigating further, Zasloff found a whole new class of antibiotics, which he christened "magainins," from the Hebrew word for shield. When isolated and tested, magainins not only killed bacteria but also destroyed some fungi, parasites, and even some tumors! Zasloff created a company—Magainin Pharmaceuticals—to bring these drugs to market.

Magainins kill bacteria in an unusual manner. Negative charges on the surface of the bacteria molecule attract the positively charged magainin. Once in place, the magainin acts like an armor-piercing cell, punching a hole in the microbe's cell wall, thereby killing the bacteria. A magainin known as pexiganin offers great promise, having successfully completed phase-2 trials for the treatment of diabetic foot ulcers, a serious infection that afflicts over one hundred thousand Americans each year. Pexiganin has not only demonstrated effectiveness in treating the ulcers but has proven its potency against some strains of drug-resistant bacteria.

Zasloff's success has touched off a flurry of research into antibiotics produced by animals. These investigations have discovered bactericidal substances in humans, deer, cows, pigs, and sharks, which offer new hope of once again gaining the upper hand in the battle against disease-causing microbes, our most ancient and implacable enemy. But magainins and other animal-derived medicines still do not provide us with our most effective weapons in this battle. These are derived from our most ancient companions and allies: microbes. Given the new technologies that allow us to understand, appreciate, and utilize microbes as never before, and given the extraordinary diversity and untapped resources that microbes represent, these tiny creatures remain the most promising source of new and effective antibiotics for the foreseeable future.

Chapter Four

DRUGS FROM
BUGS

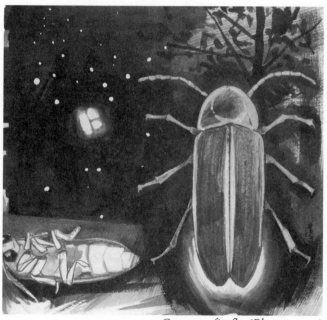

Common firefly (*Photurus sp.*)

Among terrestrial animals, none is perhaps more diversely endowed with chemical weaponry than the arthropods.

—Dr. Thomas Eisner, 1987

After having known and worked with an ancient shaman for more than a decade, I was not expecting any surprises. We were in the driest part of the dry season in that corner of the northeast Amazon, and it still felt like were hiking through a sauna. The heat seemed to suck the breath out of my body; I was bathed in sweat, and my vision had started to blur at the edges. Impervious to the scorching temperature, the old medicine man hiked on until I called ahead, asking him to pause so that I might catch my breath and take a sip of water from my canteen. A dove cooed softly in the distance as I perched on the giant trunk of a fallen *bergibita* tree and greedily gulped the precious liquid. The medicine man approached as if he too wanted a drink, but declined the proffered canteen. Instead, he snapped a small branch off the tree on which I was sitting and plunged it into an anthill nestled against the fallen trunk. Furious black ants boiled out of the nest, climbing the stick that had invaded their sanctuary. Before they could reach his hand, the shaman held the ant-encrusted branch against the inside of his left elbow. Too stunned to say anything, I watched six or seven ants bite into his flesh. He grimaced deeply and then quickly brushed them off with his right hand.

"Why—why did you do that?" I blurted out, stunned by the peculiar performance.

"Helps my arthritis," he replied, still grimacing in pain.

"But you told me you didn't use bugs as medicine, even though I asked you several times."

"Listen," he said, "we mostly use plants for healing. You know a bit about plants and I don't mind telling you about the ones most important to us. But you don't know anything about bugs, and I'm not going to waste my time teaching you!"

Similar reports of using insects to treat arthritis have filtered in from various corners of Amazonia. One enterprising Canadian pharmaceutical company took these reports seriously enough to investigate. Their findings: a heretofore unknown complex sugar molecule in the ant's venom that appears to provide temporary relief from the pain and swelling typical of arthritis.

Arthritis, a generic term for inflammation of the joints, afflicts forty million Americans (one in seven!) and hundreds of millions of people around the world. According to Dr. Robert Jacobs, a pharmacologist at the University of California at Santa Barbara and an authority on this disease, arthritis represents the leading cause of disability in the United States and annually costs the country billions in medical care and lost wages. In its more severe forms, like rheumatoid arthritis, the disease can deform and cripple a person as the joints degenerate. When cells are damaged, the human body reacts with what is known as the inflammatory response: heat, pain, redness, and swelling. This is how the body segregates and attempts to destroy injurious invaders like bacteria and viruses, or reverse harmful processes like acid burns and systemic afflictions. Because much of the damage suffered by arthritics is caused by an unremitting inflammation of the joints, one possible way to mitigate or prevent these problems would be to halt or interfere with the inflammatory response. Several factors—infections, the presence of certain enzymes, allergic reactions, and so on—can produce inflammation in the human body. Available medications offer only temporary relief from arthritis, since they treat the symptoms of the disease rather than its underlying cause.

Given current demographics, especially the aging of the baby-boom generation, the number of Americans afflicted with arthritis is expected to rise 50 percent in the next two decades. New and effective treatments for arthritis and other inflammatory disorders are a high priority on everyone's agenda. Jacobs believes natural products offer hope for finding new treatments for arthritis and is busily developing a new drug from a yellow marine sponge that blocks two different causes of the disease. The products that he is investigating show promise not only for arthritis, but also for the treatment of shock, chemical burns, and inflammatory bowel disease.

Though Jacobs focuses on marine organisms, insects and related arthropods (such as spiders and ticks, which are scientifically classified as arachnids rather than true insects) offer tremendous promise for better treatments for myriad ailments because of their astonishing species diversity and dazzling biochemical complexity. Of all the species on earth that have been classified by scientists (about 1.5 million), more than half are insects, yet we estimate that there may be more than 29 million species of arthropods that have yet to be named, much less studied.

A turning point in the relationship between the human animal and the rest of the species with which we share our planet occurred in 1982 when Smithsonian Institution entomologist Dr. Terry Erwin conducted a study that rocked the natural-history establishment. Before Erwin's groundbreaking work, scientists had estimated that the earth harbored about three million species altogether. We knew that the rain forest contained many of those species, but we were unable to ascertain how many there were. And we knew that insects comprised most of the species found there. Through an ingenious system of covering a single tree in the Peruvian Amazon with a series of nets and spraying an insecticide underneath, Erwin was able to determine exactly how many insect species lived on that tree and, by extrapolation, how many species of insects lived on our planet. So astounding were his findings, so much more diverse was the insect fauna than what he expected to find, that the estimate of insect life on earth rocketed from three million to more than thirty million species. The human species was revealed to comprise a much tinier percentage of global biodiversity than almost anyone had realized. We are vastly outnumbered!

Some scientists have taken issue with Erwin's conclusions, claiming that his estimates are too high. But exploration of the natural world, from the ocean floor to terrestrial soils to rain forest canopies, usually reveals greater diversity than previously believed. (And, as someone who has climbed into the rain forest canopy to collect plants, I can assure you that there exists no end to new species of spiders, flies, ticks, mosquitoes, and other creatures anxious to climb into your hair, drop down your shirt, drink your sweat, suck your blood, or generally make the intruding biologist feel altogether unwelcome!) As Dr. Adrian Forsyth, without question the most eloquent biologist on the subject of bugs, has pointed out, "there are hundreds, if not thousands, of specialized little mites that live only in the bills of hummingbirds, for example. Who knows exactly how many there are, what they are doing there, how they live, or what they may be good for?"

Even the figure of thirty million species doesn't quite convey the degree to which these creatures dominate our planet. University of Illinois entomologist Dr. May Berenbaum has calculated that a single termite colony can contain over a million individuals, while a locust swarm can consist of a billion individuals. She estimates that there are ten quintillion (10,000,000,000,000,000,000) insects on the planet at any time. Clearly, known species of arthropods produce many potentially therapeutic compounds. Berenbaum wrote in her delightful book *Bugs in the System:*

> When it comes to the synthesis of chemicals, insects are, as is their wont in most endeavors, tremendously prolific. Not only do they synthesize a wide assortment of their own chemicals— defensive sprays, mating and alarm pheromones, venoms and toxins—but many can incorporate into their bodies chemicals from the plants they eat. Suffice it to say that the enormous assortment of chemicals associated with insects includes compounds that are demonstrably emetic, vesicant, irritating, cardioactive, or neurotoxic—in short, the insect world is a veritable drugstore of pharmacodynamic agents.

But if this panoply of chemicals has been documented in the fewer than one million species that have already been studied, imagine what awaits in the other twenty-nine million (not to mention chemicals in the known species that have yet to be discovered)!

"Insects and their relatives," insists Dr. Thomas Eisner of Cornell University, "are the single most promising and untapped resource in terms of finding new pharmaceuticals from Mother Nature." He should know. Eisner is the leading authority on the medicinal potential of insects and their brethren. A German Jew who managed to escape the Nazis at the last possible minute, Eisner and his family fled to Uruguay, where they arrived penniless and unable to speak Spanish. Through a combination of brilliance and diligence, Eisner learned not only Spanish but English and many other skills—enough to obtain entrance to Harvard University as an undergraduate just a few years after his unpromising arrival in Uruguay. Eisner has had a long and brilliant career, publishing hundreds of papers and winning numerous awards, making him one of the most admired and influential scientists ever to have served on the Cornell faculty. Visitors to his office cannot but help be struck by two unusual sights: a piano in his laboratory (Eisner is a talented jazz pianist) and a letter from Cornell University to eighteen-year-old Thomas Eisner politely declining his request for admission to the class of 1943.

In his unique position as a European, an American, and a Latin American, Eisner has tirelessly championed the conservation cause. He has been an outspoken and influential proponent of viewing ecosystem protection (particularly rain forest conservation) as an economic opportunity rather than an economic sacrifice. Eisner played a major role in brokering a deal between Merck and the government of Costa Rica in which the pharmaceutical giant agreed to share with Costa Rica a portion of any profits derived from new drugs based on local plants and animals.

Eisner emphasizes that both the prevalence and the variety of insect species is proof of their abilities as chemical warriors. They are able to ward off predators, defeat plants' chemical defenses, and thrive from the frozen polar regions to the steaming forests of the equatorial regions.

And the unspeakable weirdness of many bugs may sometimes

indicate the presence of undreamed-of chemical compounds. In his extraordinary book *The Natural History of Sex,* Adrian Forsyth noted that male honeybees often explode after consummating their nuptial flight, and that some mites are born pregnant. There are moths in tropical Asia that suck human blood. Certain species of flea larvae actually attach their mouths to the anuses of adult fleas, thereby ensuring, as May Berenbaum wrote, "that fecal material does not go to waste."

The common bedbug ranks among the most grotesque members of the bug world. Unfazed by the female's lack of a vagina, the male bedbug plunges his organ through her abdomen and releases his sperm into the abdominal cavity. Though some of the sperm manage to find and fertilize the eggs, the female digests the remainder as a meal!

Native to Europe, the bedbug originally inhabited the lairs of large European mammals. With the global spread of *Homo sapiens* (not to mention the extinction of many species of large European mammals like the cave bear and the woolly rhinoceros), the bedbug found it much more worthwhile to concentrate its bloodsucking efforts on our species. Consequently, the bedbug has a new niche: cheap hotels and flophouses the world over, where it preys on unsuspecting and exhausted tourists (although the characteristic stench it exudes warns off the wary entomologist!).

Yet if bedbugs are in the habit of feasting on human blood, humans in turn have made excellent medical use of bedbug blood. This blood contains a hearty gumbo of chemicals and has long figured in the medicinal practices of many different cultures. As early as the first century A.D., Dioscorides was prescribing an effective treatment for some bladder problems based on roasted insects whose hemolymph contained sodium salts. Technically known as "hemolymph," insect blood is especially rich in antibacterial compounds. Dioscorides particularly valued bedbugs for the treatment of external wounds. Around the same time, Pliny was recommending headless beetles as a cure for infected wounds. Chinese texts have long included prescriptions for the use of bedbugs to treat bacterial infections like sties and infected wounds. In one account, published in 1590, a healer wrote: "In case of chronic ulceration with a gaping wound, apply locally some bedbugs, the heads of which should be removed."

Native American shamans in Amazonia have never been thought to employ many insects for medicinal purposes. Nonetheless, I believe that the dearth of data on this subject has more to do with our ignorance than their lack of knowledge: there simply aren't any full-time ethnoentomologists working in these jungles to document what local healers know and use. A Brazilian shaman that I had known for years recently shared a recipe for a concoction that he employs as a treatment "for children that cry in the night"—a tea prepared by boiling local roaches. It may be that antimicrobial compounds in the hemolymph cure a bacterial infection; it may be that the roaches' fat soothes the child's aching throat; or it may be that when Mom says, "Stop crying or I'm going to give you the roach juice!" the child becomes very quiet.

Of all the insects, perhaps the most promising group of chemical warriors is the beetles. They represent the most diverse group of insects—more than four hundred thousand species of beetles have been described by scientists, and as many as another twenty-six million have yet to be studied. Their extraordinary species diversity led the great British biologist J. B. S. Haldane to say, when asked what a life devoted to the study of biology had led him to conclude about the Creator, "He has a great fondness for beetles!" Weevils are just one of many types of beetles—and we have already described more species of weevils than there are species of mammals. Beetles thrive just about everywhere—from the Namib Desert of southern Africa to the boreal forests of northern Canada, in fresh water and in salt water, and some are even able to lay their eggs in hot springs. They eat everything—from roots to shoots, from books to dung. But the most mind-boggling aspect of beetles is their unparalleled abilities as chemical warriors.

Like some sort of entomological skunk, the *Eleodes* beetle will stand on its head when threatened and spray a stinking and odoriferous mixture at the approaching predator. The *Galerita* beetle sprays a mixture of compounds from paired glands in its abdomen. An assassin bug from Zanzibar not only injects its poisonous saliva directly into its insect prey, but also has the ability to spray it several feet in the direction of a would-be predator. The saliva contains several toxic components and bears a chemical resemblance to cobra venom.

The defense glands of many aquatic beetles brim with steroids, a class of chemicals used in a variety of medicines from birth control pills to anti-inflammatory agents. These compounds are poisonous to the fish and amphibians that prey (or attempt to prey) on these beetles. Not all beetle poisons are steroids, though. The *Ilybus fenestratus* contains an alkaloid extremely poisonous to small mammals (and we have seen how toxic compounds sometimes have medicinal potential). Another alkaloid, colymbetin, isolated from the closely related species *Colymbetes fuscus*, not only features a chemical structure unlike any other found in this group, but also functions differently: it lowers blood pressure in mammals.

The most famous—or infamous—beetle chemical occurs in the hemolymph of blister beetles. Although the technical name is cantharidin, it is more widely known as "Spanish fly," though it is not particularly Spanish and is not produced by flies. Most of it is extracted from the Eurasian metallic-blue beetle *Lytta vesicatoria*, but the compound has actually been found in over two thousand species. Spanish fly is an effective aphrodisiac—if you wish to sexually excite a female blister beetle. When a female meets a male blister beetle, she checks a gland in his head for the presence of cantharidin. According to Eisner and his colleagues, she will only mate with him if he has the chemical, which she cannot produce herself. As part of the mating ritual, the male presents her with a gift of cantharidin, which she then uses to coat her eggs.

The female covers the eggs because cantharidin has toxic properties that repel predators. Rubbed on human skin, it causes blisters, hence the name "blister beetles." The compound has been employed medicinally since Pliny's day because blistering was believed to draw out the poison. Though the lethal dose may be as little as ten milligrams, cantharidin has been used to treat many ailments, from baldness to lethargy (and is undoubtedly more effective for the latter than the former). Dermatologists still use the beetle juice to burn off several types of warts. But cantharidin has attained its greatest fame as a reputed aphrodisiac. The Marquis de Sade was prosecuted in 1772 for poisoning several prostitutes by feeding them Spanish fly–laced chocolates. Oscar Wilde was said to have also been a devotee of the drug. In a celebrated case that took more than a century to solve, French soldiers in northern Africa who dined on local frogs suffered "erections *douloureuses et prolongées*." Eisner and his colleagues fed frogs a steady diet of blister beetles for several days and then tested the amphibians, finding that they stored quantities of cantharidin in their thigh muscles sufficient to have produced the Viagra-like effects in the unfortunate Frenchmen.

Though considered "bugs" by most of the general populace, spiders differ from true insects by having eight legs and two body parts (the cephalothorax and the abdomen) rather than three. Spiders thrive on every continent except Antarctica. Primarily terrestrial creatures, several species have adapted to an aquatic life by trapping air bubbles and carrying them underwater with them, a sort of forerunner to scuba diving. Spiders are carnivores with a serious problem: they cannot eat solid food. They must capture their prey, kill it, and begin digesting it outside their body by covering the hapless creature with digestive enzymes and then slurping up the liquid.

As hunters and killers of insects, spiders have no equal. Studies in both the United States and Great Britain have confirmed that these arachnids eat a quantity of insects each year that outweighs the local human population. Dr. Michael Robinson of the National Zoo in Washington, D.C., has determined that spiders kill more insects than do either birds or commercial insecticides, and that better management of these arachnids in plantation agriculture could sharply reduce (or even eliminate, in some cases) the use of commercial pesticides.

Like cone snails, spiders often hunt, kill, and devour creatures larger than they are (one species in the Amazon feasts on small birds!). And, like cone snails, spiders have evolved powerful and deadly venoms to immobilize and kill their prey. Because of black widow spiders' well-deserved reputation as insect predators, early research focused on development of black widow venom as a commercial insecticide. The poison molecule proved complex and difficult to synthesize, so investigators initiated programs to analyze the poisons of other species and consequently stumbled onto a potential gold mine of bioactive substances. The poison of a single species may contain more than one hundred separate toxins. Kathryn Phillips wrote in *Discover* magazine:

> A single species' venom is like a massive chemistry set just waiting to be explored. . . . Researchers have found that many of the toxins are able to home in on and block key gateways in nerve cells with a precision unmatched by other substances. As a result, these toxins are proving invaluable for learning precisely how nerve cells in the brain work; they are revealing many of the chemicals and processes responsible for cell life, disease and death. Indeed, they may be the key that will one day help doctors restore health to a victim of stroke or brain seizure.

Spider venoms have already contributed to our medical system by helping us better understand our own nervous system. The initial breakthrough came in 1982 when Japanese scientists at the Tokyo Metropolitan Institute of Neuroscience studying orb-weaving spiders found that a component of their poison blocked the effects of glutamate in nerve cells. Glutamate is an amino acid that functions as a neurotransmitter, carrying messages from one nerve cell to another. Moreover, too much glutamate can destroy a nerve cell—precisely what transpires after a stroke. And an overabundance of glutamate has been implicated in some epileptic seizures. A drug that blocks glutamate without the serious side effects of other glutamate blockers offers hope for the treatment of these and other neurological problems.

Funnel-web spider venoms operate in a different way: they block calcium channels, which play a vital role in the communication between nerve cells. Research into this poison has already led to a better understanding of cerebellum function, and may in turn lead to new treatments for neurological disorders like chronic pain and paralysis. And the potential ramifications include novel treatments for diseases as dissimilar as hyperparathyroidism and osteoporosis. A pharmaceutical company in Utah is busily investigating these leads.

The spider's contribution to medicine and industry may not depend solely on its venom. Nor is a spider's ability to feed itself wholly dependent on the poison; sometimes its hunting abilities are at least as important. Spitting spiders are but one example; when flies make the mistake of getting too close, the spider quickly emits two crisscrossing strands of saliva impregnated with venom that both pins and kills the hapless prey. An even more diabolical hunter is the bola spider, who produces a substance that smells similar to the odor of female moths in heat. The spider then tips a strand of its own silk with a tiny drop of a gluelike substance. As the bewildered male moth flies by looking for love, the cowboyesque arachnid whirls the strand and throws the glue-tipped end at the insect. Unlike the cowboy, the spider can lasso its prey in the dark!

Spiders also employ disguises to get close enough to administer their venom. Some tropical species are astounding ant mimics: like ants, they have three body segments instead of the usual two. To take this entomological species-transvestism one step further, they walk on six legs, holding the other two legs over their heads like antennae. When an unsuspecting ant meets one of these undercover spiders and hold out its antennae to communicate, it receives a fatal bite instead of a reassuring signal.

Thousands of years ago, healers noted that cobwebs placed in a wound hasten coagulation. Pliny (ca. A.D. 79) recorded this in ancient Rome, and spiderwebs are still employed for the same purpose in rural Italy and many other countries. Some debate exists as to whether cobwebs contain antimicrobial compounds. Their effectiveness is probably due to the webbing's serving as a structure on which the blood clots begin to form.

Cobwebs were employed as bombsight crosshairs during the Second World War and are still used in surveying instruments and telescopic gunsights. In an age when new materials are constantly being invented, cobwebs remain one of the toughest and most resilient materials known, being both softer than cotton yet several times stronger than steel. Engineer Nick Ashley, an authority on cobwebs, noted that "a fly hitting a spider web is like a fighter jet flying into a piece of fishing net, yet the web absorbs the impact and stops the fly dead."

These unique attributes of cobwebs have caught the eye of both industry and the military. Even though a single spider can produce over a hundred feet of silk in a day, it is still not enough to make commercial development feasible. Enter the biotech engineers: they are implanting the genes of the spider that code for the production of cobwebs into bacteria, and these microorganisms are beginning to produce silk molecules. Many hurdles still have to be overcome before the scientists can generate silk. One of their many questions is why industry requires high temperature and powerful solvents to produce exceedingly durable materials when spiders can create cobwebs with water at room temperature.

Once artificial spider silk can be produced commercially (and it will happen in the not too distant future), the military will be using it to make lightweight aircraft, bulletproof vests, parachute cords, and satellites. And medical personnel will be using it to produce artificial heart valves, membranes, tendons, veins, skin, and nonallergenic sutures.

Like spiders, fireflies produce chemicals with medicinal potential—Eisner and his colleagues isolated antiviral and cardiac stimulants from these flying insects—as well as compounds with medical applications. Remember the so-called Golden Fleece Awards given by Senator William Proxmire, from 1975 to 1988, to what he considered the most egregious and wasteful spending of government funding? The award recipient was often some poor researcher engaged in so-called pure research, that is, with no immediate industrial application. Adrian Forsyth suggests that it might be better to remember the award as a testimony to the degree of ignorance at the highest levels of decision making. One recipient of Proxmire's award was a scientist who began studying firefly communication biology and luminescence and, in so doing, helped provide us with a weapon against one of humanity's deadliest afflictions.

With the possible exception of malaria, tuberculosis has probably killed more people than any other single disease. In the 1940s, Dr. Selman Waksman and his colleagues from Rutgers University developed streptomycin from a soil mold, the first known cure for the deadly ailment. Streptomycin-resistant strains soon arose and were all but extirpated by additional medications developed by Gerhard Domagk in Germany and Jorgen Lehmann in Denmark. When the three drugs were used together, the cure rate approached 100 percent.

Thirty years later, however, tuberculosis has returned in a more frightening form. The disease is not only reappearing in U.S. urban centers, but it is spreading throughout Africa, where it never really disappeared. TB has become the number one cause of death in people with damaged immune systems. Medical personnel around the world are frightened: multiple drug resistance among the tuberculosis bacillus has become increasingly common. A major obstacle to effective treatment: TB is such a slow-growing organism that it can take up to three months for doctors to determine if the patient has contracted a drug-resistant strain—and, meanwhile, the bacteria continue to spread in the patient's body. By using a light-generating reaction catalyzed by an enzyme of the firefly, doctors can reduce screening time to just a few days. When a proper drug mixture is added to the petri dish, the lights dim.

The firefly test is by no means limited to tuberculosis. It serves as a rapid and effective test for contamination by microbes. If researching bugs and other natural products doesn't seem financially feasible, consider this: The Coca-Cola Company uses a version of the firefly test to screen sodas before they are bottled. Last year, Coke paid the U.S. government many millions of dollars in taxes—

quite a bit more money than the government had given in grant funds to the scientist whose research led to the use of firefly enzymes in medicine and industry.

Ants, as we saw with the shaman at the beginning of the chapter, have a history in the medical field as well as the potential to make a future contribution. The giant army ant of the American tropics is often featured in rain forest documentaries and even served as the "heavy" in a Charlton Heston B movie in the 1950s. Hundreds of thousands of army ants swarming through a tropical forest, accompanied by antbirds swooping down and gobbling up insects flushed by the approaching ant army, is one of nature's most unforgettable spectacles.

Though famous for their militaristic marching behavior, they are also employed by Indians of the northeast Amazon for an unusual medical purpose: to stitch wounds. The edges of the wound are manually pinched together and a soldier ant is held to the laceration and encouraged to bite (not that it needs much encouragement!). If positioned correctly, the ant sinks its fishhook-shaped mandibles into the two edges of the wound, holding them together. The body of the ant is then twisted off, killing the insect. Because the muscles that close the jaws are stronger than those that open them, the suture remains in place. Similar practices have been documented in both Africa and Asia.

An innovative approach to finding new therapeutics among the ants entails what Australian entomologist Dr. Andrew J. Beattie terms "biorational deduction." He wrote:

> It is time to explore the possibility that better deployment of the biological sciences can significantly increase the probability of success. In fact, the exploration for and the discovery of new bioresources should become a challenging biological discipline in its own right. . . . The basic premise of such a discipline is that because we share the environment of Earth with millions of species, we and the other species have many problems in common. Problems solved by other species over millions of

years of natural selection may provide, or point to, solutions useful to us.

Beattie utilizes this approach in a search for novel antibiotics. He reasoned that antibiotic substances are likely to have evolved where the problem of contagion is most common. Most creatures, from elephants to penguins, spend at least part of their existence living with other members of their species. But social insects like wasps, bees, and ants live in closest proximity to each other, thus increasing their potential susceptibility to infectious disease.

Ants produce several antibiotic substances from their metapleural glands. These compounds are used to suppress fungal and bacterial growth in the ants' nests. A most extraordinary application has been documented in the insidious fire ant, a native of South America that has been moving north into the United States for several decades. Workers guarding the "nursery" extrude and vibrate their stingers over the brood, producing an antibiotic aerosol that, believes entomologist Dr. William Vander Meer of the U.S. Department of Agriculture, protects the little ones from microorganisms. Enormous amounts of aerosol are sprayed elsewhere to repel other ant species. Similar behavior, in which much greater amounts of venom are dispensed, dissuades other species of ants from entering the nest. This fumigant, only recently documented, explains why ancient cultures valued what they called "medicated earth"—which consisted mostly of old ant nests.

The honeybee—ubiquitous, common, taken for granted—represents both the promise and the peril facing the development of novel insect-derived therapies. Although the species with which we are most familiar is the common honeybee (originally native to Europe), scientists estimate there may be as many as forty thousand different species of bees, ranging in size from the two-inch black giant to the tiny panurgine bee, which is less than one-tenth of an inch long. Despite these 39,999 other species, it is the honeybee that has long served *Homo sapiens* as a sort of flying pharmacy.

Honeybee venom has proven to be complex mixtures of powerful chemicals, some with proven therapeutic capabilities. Hippocrates himself noted how people suffering from ailments such as arthritis often experienced relief from the pain and inflammation after a bee sting. Bee venom contains more than ten active compounds. Holistic physician Glenn Rothfeld relies on bee venom therapy (BVT) to alleviate the pain and swelling associated with both rheumatoid arthritis and osteoarthritis. Other types of non-joint inflammations (such as asthma and ulcerative colitis) have also shown improvement in some cases.

Many acute and chronic injuries—bursitis, tendonitis, chronic neck and back pain, for example—often respond well to BVT, according to Rothfeld. Some healers are even using bee stings as a nonsurgical alternative to improving the appearance of keloids and other unattractive scar tissue, since BVT partially dissolves and softens the scar tissue so it not only flattens out but fades in color.

By far the most controversial therapeutic application of BVT is in the treatment of multiple sclerosis (MS). This crippling disease is caused when the immune system attacks the myelin sheaths surrounding the nerves, causing blindness, loss of sensation and coordination, and, eventually, death. BVT does not cure MS but seems effective at relieving many of the symptoms.

People suffering from fatal diseases for which there is no known cure are (understandably) willing to try almost anything, making them notoriously susceptible to unscrupulous types peddling remedies that are both expensive and ineffective. Jane Brody of the *New York Times* lambasted BVT in a 1993 column subtitled "Folk Medicine versus Good Science," as if there could be no overlap between the two (hasn't she ever taken an aspirin?). She correctly pointed out that bee stings can cause fatal reactions, although this is rare and is carefully monitored by bee venom therapists. Brody also correctly noted that laboratory studies of BVT were needed to qualify and quantify its effectiveness. So compelling are the numerous testimonials to the effectiveness of BVT by MS sufferers, however, that the Multiple Sclerosis Society recently gave a grant to the Thomas Jefferson Medical College in Philadelphia to investigate BVT in a clinical setting.

Bee venom packs a multifaceted therapeutic punch because of its potent chemicals. About half the poison in a honeybee's sting consists of melittin, which is highly antibacterial and efficacious in treating some varieties of both gram-positive and gram-negative bacteria.

Still another therapeutic component of the venom is adolapin, which functions as both a painkiller and an anti-inflammatory. An additional anti-inflammatory is apamin, which enhances nerve transmission and is believed to be a mood elevator (this would explain why some claim to "feel better" after being stung). Mast cell degranulating peptide (usually referred to by the abbreviation MCDP) is said to rival the effectiveness of hydrocortisone as an anti-inflammatory agent. Hyaluronidase comprises a small part of bee venom and is found in other insect venoms as well. It is believed to augment the permeability of the tissue at the sting site, thus enhancing blood flow, providing some relief and facilitating the uptake of other venom components into the bloodstream.

In his best-selling book *Spontaneous Healing,* the Harvard-trained physician and holistic healer Dr. Andrew Weil described a most extraordinary case in which a bee sting played a pivotal role. Weil tells the tale of Oliver W., an eighty-six-year-old man who had suffered severe rheumatoid arthritis for almost thirty years. The poor fellow was consuming twelve aspirin a day to manage the persistent pain. After trying a multitude of different medicines and therapies without success, he assumed that a successful treatment did not exist. Then a most extraordinary event transpired:

On this particular day, my wife had washed my pajamas and hung them out on the clothesline to dry. When dry, they were folded and put on the bed. I retired at 10 P.M. and put them on. About 1:30 A.M. I got up to go to the bathroom and felt a sting on the inside of my left knee. I slapped it hard, shook my leg and out fell a honeybee. Two days later the bee sting was still swollen and sore, but the arthritis swelling in that knee began to go down. The next day, the pain from the sting subsided, and I stopped taking the extra-strength aspirin, because the pain and swelling in all my joints began to recede. Two weeks later, I stopped all the medication. Within five or six weeks, the swelling and inflammation were gone from all the joints. I've never been bothered by arthritis since.

As Weil pointed out, the patient did not undergo true apitherapy. This would have entailed multiple stings over a period long enough for the chemicals in the venom to gradually cure his condition. The venom components injected during a single sting are usually insufficient to effect a cure. Weil hypothesizes that the single sting Oliver received somehow "changed the dynamics of an autoimmune problem of long-standing, activating a complete and permanent healing response."

Beeswax has long been a standard ingredient in medical ointments, plasters, and even suppositories. Two other bee-related products—bee pollen and propolis—are sold in almost every health food store, despite the fact that laboratory analysis indicates that at least some of the sterling qualities attributed to them are usually overstated. Bee pollen is a mixture of bee saliva, plant nectar, and pollen that can consist of up to 30 percent protein and contains amino acids, carotenes, sugars, and vitamins (all of these substances can be purchased cheaper if bought separately). Propolis, which does exhibit antibiotic properties and was employed in wound dressings during the Boer War, can only marginally be considered a "bee product" since it is actually produced by the buds of coniferous trees. The bees collect the material and carry it back home, where it is mostly used to caulk cracks in the hive. Propolis also has another use: when an uninvited visitor (such as a mouse in search of honey) invades the hive, the enraged bees mount a furious defense and sting it to death. If the carcass is too large for the bees to push out of the hive, they cover it with propolis. Instead of rotting, the corpse eventually mummifies. Physician Guido Majno has suggested that this mummification process can be attributed to the dry atmosphere within the hive, but the antibiotic components of the propolis prevent putrefaction.

Honey has proven to be a more effective bee-derived medicine than propolis. Most inhabitants of the industrialized world cannot comprehend the enormous roles honey sometimes assumes in tribal societies. The Akuriyos are a small band of semi-nomadic Amerindians with whom I have worked since the mid-1980s. Inhabiting the remote forests of the Brazil-Suriname border region, they did not come into sustained contact with the outside world until about twenty years ago. Because they had no agriculture, they did not have access to sugar cane, which, although it was introduced into the Amazon from tropical Asia only four hundred years ago, is found in almost every Amerindian garden in tropical America. Consequently, they were (and still are) obsessed with honey. The Akuriyos have more than twenty words for honey. The second major cause of death among adult males (after jaguar attacks) was falling out of trees while searching for beehives. I have often set off with the Akuriyos in search of healing plants, only to have them disappear into the forest with a happy shout when they heard the telltale buzzing of bees from some distant tree. Though most of the honey is devoured on the spot as an Amazonian version of carbo-loading, a portion is often carefully wrapped in a palm leaf and carried back to the village both for future consumption and for healing purposes.

Honey's medicinal properties were extolled in Sumerian tablets carved four thousand years ago; honey also served as the most widely used drug in ancient Egypt, appearing in more than half the remedies in surviving accounts. Though honey was used for just about every malady imaginable, the Egyptians often employed it for the treatment of burns, wounds, and other bacteria-related ailments. Despite modern medicine's relative lack of interest in honey, it has proven to be a highly effective antibacterial compound. Honey's most effective mode of action (due to its high sugar content) is its ability to draw water out of the bacterial cells, causing them to shrink and die. Because this destroys the bacteria by a different method than that of antibiotics like penicillin, honey is not only widely employed in the more remote corners of the world as an anti-infective agent, it is also being evaluated as a treatment for certain strains of drug-resistant bacteria.

And, because of its ability to draw water out of cells and repel bacteria, honey has also been used on occasion as an embalming fluid. When a Maccabean king of Israel was poisoned, Marc Antony had the body preserved in honey until it could be carried back to Jerusalem, where it could be given a proper burial, according to the chronicles of Josephus. And when Alexander the Great died of malaria during his campaign to conquer India, his body was packed in honey and returned to Egypt.

Although honey's use as a wound dressing never truly disappeared, it was not until the mid-1940s that its effectiveness was confirmed in the lab. However, spurred on by the development of penicillin and other fungi-derived drugs for the war effort, the "antibiotic revolution" was in full swing. The pharmaceutical companies focused their efforts on marketing these drugs (which consumers could not produce in backyard beehives). Consequently, honey never became part of the antibacterial armentarium employed by today's physicians.

This may be about to change. A spate of recent publications has highlighted the successful use of honey to treat infected wounds and burns that do not respond well to conventional treatment. A recent editorial in the *Journal of the Royal Society of Medicine* stated, "The time has come for conventional medicine to lift the blinds off this traditional remedy and give it its due recognition."

Both the bee's sting and its honey have served our species as curative agents for thousands of years. Once again, however, new technologies augment this potential even further. The Canadian firm Micrologix Biotech is developing a new class of antibiotics based on chemicals found in insects. By fusing melittin from the honeybee with another peptide—cecropin from the giant silkworm moth—they have produced an entirely new class of antibiotics. Using genetic engineering and combinatorial chemistry, scientists then create more potent varieties using the original fused compound as the basepoint.

These new "bug drugs" function differently from many fungi-derived antibiotics, so they prove useful complements for treating drug-resistant bacteria. Penicillin, for example, interferes with the ability of bacteria to build cell walls necessary for bacterial growth and reproduction. But like armor-piercing cells, the bug drugs bind to bacterial cell walls and punch holes in them, killing the bacteria. As laboratory research continues, antibiotics from bees, moths, and other bugs may add to our store of antibiotic medications.

The medical potential of the insects and their relatives has barely been tapped. But as science and the pharmaceutical industry have begun to investigate, the resource has started to diminish. Consider what is happening to the honeybee, a microcosm of what is happening in the world at large. The honeybee's major economic importance right now is not medical but agricultural. According to bee biologist Dr. Steve Buchmann and ethnobotanist Dr. Gary Nabhan, a staggering 15 percent of U.S. food crops are wholly dependent on honeybees for pollination. In other words, no bees, no pollination, no soybeans, no cowpeas, no chickpeas, no broadbeans, no almonds, no mustard, no cabbage, no cucumbers, no chili peppers, no eggplants, no oranges, no watermelons, no tangerines, no lemons, no limes, no grapefruits, no melons, no peaches, no plums, no strawberries, no apricots, and no cherries. Buchmann and Nabhan point out that, during the past fifty years, the number of managed bee colonies in the United States has declined by 50 percent due to disease, pesticide poison, competition with Africanized bees, and misguided government agricultural policies. Imagine what has happened with nonmanaged populations, which, in some cases, are more susceptible to these factors. And imagine what sort of healing compounds are to be found in these other species, virtually all of which are less well known in terms of their venom—and their healing potential—than are the common honeybees.

Chapter Five

HIDEOUS
HEALERS

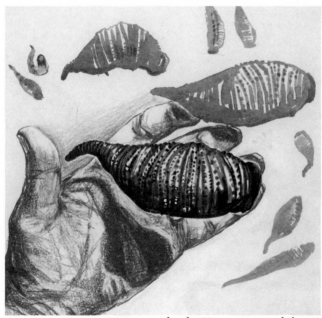

Amazonian leech (*Haementaria ghilianii*)

Secretions from bloodsucking animals are to cardiovascu-
lar diseases what penicillin is to infectious diseases.

—Dr. Roy Sawyer, 1994

In June 1987, I landed in South America in search of an endangered species of man-eating crocodilian.

The black caiman, once widespread and common in tropical
South America, had been extinguished from much of its former
range, mostly by hunters in search of the reptiles' lustrous black-
and-yellow hide. I'd heard reports of an enormous population of
these crocodilians thriving in a swampy backwater of French
Guiana, itself something of a colonial backwater, situated in the
northeast shoulder of South America. A colleague and I hired a local Creole by the name of Georges to take us up the Kaw River,
whose upper reaches were said to be inhabited by these reptilian
throwbacks to the age of the dinosaurs.

Wearing only an Australian bush hat and a tiny red bathing
suit almost invisible beneath a sizable paunch, Georges cut a memorable figure standing in the back of the motorized dugout canoe as
we entered the mouth of the river. The emerald forest that lined
both banks was barely visible through the early morning mist. Going against the current and fueled by a tiny outboard engine, we
made slow progress as the increasing heat of the equatorial sun
burned off the haze. I caught a quick glimpse of a sunbittern before
the bird hid itself in the riverside vegetation; in the sky above us
black-headed vultures cruised in search of carrion. The forest
seemed unnaturally quiet while the water was as still as glass. For a
fleeting moment, I felt as if I were a human sacrifice being sent upriver to propitiate the caiman gods. It made my flesh crawl.

To ease my nervousness, I tried to make conversation with Georges, though he was a man of few words.

"Do you see many black caimans here?" I asked him.

"You don't *see* them, but they are here," he said, nonchalantly. This seemed to be the end of the conversation.

A few minutes of silence, then Georges spoke again.

"Of course," he added, "caimans are not the *worst* things in this river."

Puzzled, I half-turned around and asked him what he meant. "What could be worse than giant caimans?" I queried.

"Giant caiman *leeches*," he replied, wrinkling his nose and furrowing his brow to emphasize his loathing and disgust.

Georges's opinion of leeches is shared by most of our species. One of the most horrifying and unforgettable scenes in a feature film appears in John Huston's 1952 classic *The African Queen*. Humphrey Bogart, as down-on-his-luck boat captain Charlie Allnut, has had to jump into the river to haul his craft through a thick clump of reeds. He emerges from the water, saying, "If there is anything in the world I hate, it's *leeches*—filthy little devils!" As he climbs back into the boat, the camera pulls back to reveal his body covered with leeches.

Leeches are not, however, restricted to the tropics. Scientists estimate that there are 650 species of leeches; they can be found in desert water holes, oceans of the polar regions, and even on some mountains at ten thousand feet. Although most are aquatic, several species are terrestrial. Leeches feed on everything from fish to penguins to earthworms, their closest living relatives. Although most are innocuous to human health, some have proven lethal. Leeches can drink five times their weight in blood and triple their size during this process. Their appetite had a devastating effect on Napoleon's unsuspecting troops in the Middle East. Though the French conquered much of Europe, they proved no match for the gruesome attack by these invertebrates. Having completed the conquest of Egypt, Napoleon marched his troops east through the Sinai Desert in search of new territories to conquer. Parched by the desert sun, the desperate soldiers drank deeply from every water hole they passed. Some of these ponds harbored tiny leeches, which were ingested with the water. Once inside, the leeches attached themselves to the mouths and throats of the soldiers and began to feed off them. Some of the men were killed by the loss of blood but, relatively speaking, they were luckier than many of their comrades. As the leeches began to swell with blood, they blocked the throats and nasal passages of the other soldiers, who died of asphyxiation.

Despite these particularly grisly deaths, the use of leeches for therapeutic purposes is at least as old as the earliest accounts of recorded medicine. Leeches were employed by the ancient Egyptians, Greeks, Romans, Indians, and Chinese. The tomb of the Egyptian scribe Userhat (from the Eighteenth Dynasty, 1567–1308 B.C.) contains a wall painting that seems to depict a healer applying leeches to a patient. An ancient Indian text of two thousand years ago includes such detailed information on the leeches employed that twelve of the species mentioned can be identified. The noted physician Galen (A.D. 129–199) was a major figure in promulgating a theory of health based on the correct balance of the four "humors" (blood, phlegm, black bile, and yellow bile). Leeches were believed to suck out the bad blood, making them necessary for treatment of an extraordinary range of diseases. Not only were leeches applied to relieve everything from headaches to heart problems, but they were also applied to stop bleeding!

In the Middle Ages, barbers began carrying out a variety of bloodletting activities (including the application of leeches) in addition to cutting hair and trimming beards. These barber-surgeons (as they came to be called) advertised by wrapping bloody bandages on a post outside their shops. This is the origin of the barbers' pole, which still features the red-and-white spirals.

Ironically, the use of leeches for their blood-sucking abilities reached its zenith under François-Joseph Broussais, a military surgeon in Napoleon's army. Broussais believed that many diseases were caused by inflammation, and that the way to relieve inflammation was to apply leeches and plenty of them. He practiced what he preached, sometimes applying more than sixty leeches at a time to his own body. In one memorable instance, he applied fifty to sixty leeches to himself on fifteen occasions within eighteen days— to treat a case of indigestion!

Spurred on by the exhortations of Broussais, the French are estimated to have imported over a billion of the creatures during the nineteenth century—and they employed these *in addition to the leeches that were collected locally.* In the year 1833, France imported more than forty million leeches. Germany alone was reported to be importing more than thirty million a year. As demand increased, so did prices, so some pharmacies began to "rent" leeches. This movement of the creatures from one patient to another undoubtedly spread disease. Because of this extraordinary demand, as well as the decline of frog populations that are the staple food of the baby leeches, leeches became extinct over much of their original range and several countries passed laws protecting them. William Wordsworth made note of their decline in his poem "The Leech Gatherer":

> He with a smile then did his words repeat;
> And said that, gathering leeches, far and wide
> He traveled; stirring thus about with his feet
> The waters of the pool where they abide.
> Once I could meet with them on every side;
> But they have dwindled long by slow decay;
> Yet I still persevere and find them where I may.

Leeches were also employed for medical purposes in the United States. More than one million leeches were used annually between 1865 and 1915, and the most common species was a local one (*Macrobdella decora*) although the European leech was also imported. In the waning years of the nineteenth century, when the work of Pasteur and his colleagues demonstrated that microorganisms, rather than "humors" or "bad blood," usually caused disease, leeching began to decline in popularity.

These early "leech-doctors" had many misguided and incorrect notions, but were correct in believing that leeches have an effect on the way blood behaves—more correct than they could have imagined. After all, bloodsuckers have been in the hematology business many millions of years longer than hematologists, pharmacologists, and pharmaceutical companies. No wonder some of our best drugs to fight heart disease, circulatory disorders, clotting problems, and other matters of the heart are being developed from hideous healers.

The early physicians and bloodletters were also correct in believing that blood plays a crucial role in maintaining health. Blood has many vital functions in the body—it carries and circulates oxygen and carts away waste products. Blood must also be able to clot—otherwise we would all bleed to death after a simple pinprick, much like a tire that has sprung a leak. The flip side of the equation, however, is that when blood clots spontaneously, life-threatening situations may result. If heart disease causes arteries to narrow, clots sometimes form, halting the flow of blood and leading to a heart attack. Deep vein thrombosis (formation of a blood clot in the leg veins) can lead to pulmonary embolism (the blood clot lodges in the lungs), which can then cause a heart attack, a scenario that kills over one hundred thousand Americans each year. Clots forming in the brain can cause strokes, leaving the unfortunate individual impaired if not dead. Strokes are the leading cause of disability among the elderly and the number two cause of dementia (after Alzheimer's). Of the five hundred thousand Americans who suffer a stroke each year, one hundred thousand die within a month, forty-eight thousand will die within a year, and thirty thousand will suffer another stroke within the next twelve months.

Thromboembolic diseases (heart attacks and strokes) kill more people in the industrialized world than any other category of disease. *Business Week* magazine estimated that the market for anticoagulant and thrombolytic blood thinners in the United States alone was 700 million dollars in 1993 and is expected to rise to 1.1 billion dollars by the year 2000.

It is the extremely complex way in which blood does (or doesn't) clot that is (literally) at the heart of these medical problems. Blood does not clot like water freezes. Clotting entails a series of complicated and interrelated steps technically known as the "coagulation cascade," one of the most complex processes in the human body. Genentech biochemist Dr. Robert Lazarus described the sequence of events:

> To understand the mechanism of blood clotting, we have to un-
> derstand that blood clots are made up of two primary compo-
> nents—platelets and fibrin. When an injury occurs, platelets
> are first on the scene. They are activated and adhere to the in-
> jured blood-vessel wall. The activated platelets then bind fi-
> brinogen and aggregate to form a "platelet plug." Clotting
> factors are also activated, initiating the "coagulation cascade," a
> complex series of reactions which result in eventual formation
> of a blood clot. The coagulation cascade involves the conversion
> of an inactive blood protein called "prothrombin" into active
> "thrombin." Thrombin then acts as an enzyme to convert fi-
> brinogen into fibrin molecules. Fibrin monomers polymerize to
> form "thread-like" fibrin polymers. These polymers are cross-
> linked to form a matrix that traps platelets and other cells, thus
> forming a stable blood clot.

In the 1930s, scientists developed the first commercial anticoagulant: heparin, a complex carbohydrate (sugar) found in many cells
(today it is commercially extracted from cows and pigs). Heparin
impedes clotting by interfering with the coagulation cascade at
three key points: by decreasing the availability of thrombin, by preventing the formation of prothrombin, and by preventing the formation of fibrin. It is inexpensive and, in many cases, highly
effective. In a few cases, however, it causes a hideous and crippling
allergic reaction, and it was precisely this reaction that almost killed
my friend Charley. Not too long after he finished his degree at Harvard, he developed a fatal form of cancer. To thin his blood prior to
giving him an experimental drug, the doctors had administered
heparin. The result was a disaster.

Charley had an unusual reaction to the anticoagulant. His
blood platelet count declined and then clots began to form through-

out his body. What the physicians needed to do was administer an anticoagulant, but the most effective anticoagulant they had was what may have caused the clotting in the first place. Apparently, there was little they could do. A few days later, his body was covered in burnlike lesions, and they had amputated most of his fingers and toes.

The difficulty in being involved in drug development is knowing that you will eventually learn of new therapies or compounds that might have helped a friend or a relative. A new drug that only now is entering the marketplace might have prevented some of Charley's suffering. The drug is called lepirudin (Refludan), and it was developed from leeches.

One of the reasons that leeches caught the eye of early healers is the peculiar nature of wounds caused by their bites. Whereas a small puncture of the skin may bleed for a few minutes, a leech bite may ooze for ten hours. In 1884, J. B. Haycraft of the Welsh National School of Medicine published a landmark paper identifying the medical world's first anticoagulant, extracted from the saliva of the leech. It later became known as hirudin, after the scientific name of the European leech *Hirudo medicinalis*.

It wasn't until the 1950s that hirudin was first isolated by the German chemist Fritz Markwardt and thus made available in a purified form for scientific study. Hirudin soon proved invaluable in helping scientists better understand the coagulation cascade. Hirudin bonds to the thrombin, thus preventing fibrinogen from changing into fibrin, thereby preventing clots from forming. It is more effective in this sense than heparin, which binds to antithrombin III, which then inhibits thrombin. Not only is it more potent, but, unlike heparin, it does not require the presence of certain chemicals (called "cofactors") in the blood to function as an anticoagulant.

Hirudin proved twice as effective as heparin in preventing blood clots in the legs of patients who have just had hip replacements and other surgeries. The leech-derived compound also seems to lead to fewer cardiac complications than does heparin. The problem with the medical use of hirudin quickly became one of supply:

leeches were disappearing in the wild and had been placed on the endangered species list. The supply had declined yet the demand was rising sharply.

Into the picture stepped Dr. Roy Sawyer, widely recognized as the leading authority on leeches. Sawyer grew up in South Carolina, where even as a child he was fascinated with these bizarre creatures. He went on to write the three-volume book *Leech Biology and Behavior,* which, though it won't be made into a feature film in the near future, is to leech studies what the Bible is to Christianity and the Torah is to Judaism. Seeing the burgeoning demand for leeches in the medical field and the diminishing populations of these creatures in the wild, Sawyer started a business in 1984 devoted to propagating them. Sawyer christened the company Biopharm, and also coined the company's motto: "The Biting Edge of Science."

Once again, biotechnology was able to assist Mother Nature: by implanting leech DNA in bacteria, scientists have coaxed the bacteria into producing an artificial version of hirudin known as lepirudin, or Refludan. The FDA approved this drug in March of 1988 for the specific treatment of heparin-induced thrombocytopenia (which may have contributed to the suffering of my friend Charley). And there are indications that Refludan (or closely related leech-derived compounds) may also prove useful for the treatment of other thromboembolic diseases like deep vein thrombosis, unstable angina, and certain types of heart attacks.

Even though the new medicine is produced by genetic engineering, however, leeches still offer other potential benefits for future human welfare: these slimy worms are much more than merely sources of a single anticoagulant. Because the bite of these creatures is painless, leeches are believed to contain an anesthetic that allows the leech to feed undetected and thus undisturbed (one species is able to plunge a six-inch bloodsucking proboscis into your flesh without causing any pain!), yet this compound has yet to be isolated and identified. Leeches also produce substances that function as "vasodilators," which enlarge the host's blood vessels near the leech bite and thus increase blood flow into the maw of the parasite. Leech saliva has also yielded an antibiotic as well as a substance potentially useful in the treatment of glaucoma.

Roy Sawyer's comparison of the potential medical benefits of blood-sucking animals to penicillin was not hyperbole. Research on lesser-known species of leeches is uncovering numerous anticoagulant compounds that interrupt the coagulation cascade in different ways, unlike that of hirudin—meaning that *every species of leech offers the possibility of providing us with new drugs for or lessons about blood disorders and other ailments.* Dr. Robert Lazarus of Genentech studied the North American leech *Macrobdella decora* and found just what he expected: an anticoagulant compound similar in structure to hirudin. What he and his colleagues *did not* expect to find was that this compound, decorsin, would disrupt the clotting cascade in a completely different manner!

This unquestionably demonstrates the utilitarian value of biodiversity: Because every species is different, each may harbor unique compounds that can somehow benefit humankind. If we have an effective anticoagulant in heparin, why do we need Refludan? As we have seen, some people who are allergic to heparin may be helped by lepirudin. Many medical conditions can impede the clotting cascade, from blood poisoning to cancer, from snakebite to liver dysfunction. Each ailment may interfere differently with blood clotting, hence the need for a variety of anticoagulants that function in distinct ways. Furthermore, different people respond to the same doses of the same drug in dissimilar ways. The greater the variety of healing potions available, the greater the likelihood of an effective treatment free of side effects.

In 1975, Sawyer stumbled across a one-hundred-year-old paper published in Italian that described a new species of leech based on a single specimen collected near the mouth of the Amazon River. He had difficulty believing what he read: according to the publication, the leech *reached a length of eighteen inches,* making it the longest leech in the world! Excited by this lead, he combed the literature, seeking confirmation of the existence of the giant leech. Sawyer hit paydirt in an article published by a French scientist in 1899. The paper noted that the leech was not restricted to Brazil but also occurred to the northwest in French Guiana. So gigantic and blood-thirsty was this species, wrote the Frenchman, that "a few [of them] are sufficient to kill a cow or a horse."

Scientists recognize two basic types of leeches: the jawed species that bite into their prey using their teeth, and the proboscis leeches that pierce their prey with a syringelike organ through which they suck the host's blood. Because these two groups are not closely related, and because the European leech had been well-studied, Sawyer hypothesized that the giant Amazon leech might harbor new therapeutic compounds. During an arduous expedition into the mosquito-ridden marshes of French Guiana, Sawyer was able to collect thirty-five of the leeches to bring back to the lab. Within four years, he had raised ten thousand individuals from the original stock. Most importantly, his hypothesis proved correct: research at Temple University in Philadelphia revealed that the main anticoagulant was an unusual new compound, which they named hementin. Unlike hirudin, which prevents clots from coalescing, hementin *dissolves clots after they have formed!* Sawyer now refers to hementin as "the clot-buster." Hementin has the potential to dissolve platelet-rich blood clots, a type of clot relatively impervious to other drugs. It offers promise as treatment not only for cardiovascular diseases, but also arthritis and glaucoma. And another anticoagulant from this species (which functions differently from hementin!) has been isolated and is also being evaluated.

The more species of leeches we study, the more new, unusual, and potentially useful compounds we find. Eglin, from the common European leech, blocks inflammation caused by localized trauma (like surgery) and shows promise as a novel treatment for ulcerous conditions of the intestines such as Crohn's disease. New anticoagulants are also being discovered, like antistatin from a Mexican leech, and ornatin, which blocks fibrinogen binding and inhibits platelet aggregation. Evolution has provided the leech—and us—with an extraordinary panoply of different compounds, offering us new ways to study and inhibit coagulation with unlimited potential for the successful treatment of blood-related ailments.

Other bloodsucking animals offer potential treatments for

other circulatory problems. Tick anticoagulant peptide (TAP) from a bloodsucking tick and a compound from hookworm saliva each inhibit the clotting cascade by interfering with the process as soon as it is initiated, even earlier than hirudin. But the search for new anticoagulants is not limited to invertebrates or snake venoms: one company has been working on a compound found in the saliva of the vampire bat, said to be able to destroy clots that clog arteries without inducing general bleeding. The bat-derived substance has been code-named "draculin." Pharmacologist Ryan Huxtable wrote: "[On more than once occasion] insignificant species held to be of little account in one age can quickly become of economic and scientific importance. The lesson is . . . that, because we have not yet found a particular species to be of significance to us, we [cannot] conclude that it will never be of significance and can safely drive it into extinction for the sake of a temporary economic advantage."

And these creatures (and others) may prove useful in more than one medical area. Leeches now play a vital role in reattachment microsurgery, in which severed body parts (usually fingers) that have been accidentally amputated (usually in industrial mishaps) are sewn onto the patient. Typically, microsurgeons can successfully reconnect arteries, which are larger and more robust than veins. As a result, blood travels into the reattached part unimpeded. The veins however, are not as quick to resume function, so blood that finds its way into the finger may be unable to depart.

In 1985, a five-year-old Massachusetts boy was attacked by a German shepherd that bit off his right ear. At Boston's Children's Hospital, Dr. Joseph Upton surgically reattached the ear. The operation proved successful but problems ensued. The blood flowed into the ear, but clots formed in the veins, preventing the blood from exiting. The injection of anticoagulants failed to solve the problem. Fortunately, Upton had served as a military physician in Vietnam, where he had heard that leeches might solve this problem. Managing to obtain several of the creatures, he allowed them to attach themselves to the swollen and discolored areas near the ear, where they drained off the excess blood and injected anticoagulants that prevented further clotting. The leeches applied to the reattached ear served as a safety valve, sucking out the excess blood until the veins healed themselves. The maneuver proved successful and has become standard operating procedure for the reattachment of severed fingers, toes, noses, scalps, and other body parts. Biopharm serves as the world's leading breeder and supplier of medicinal leeches. Fully two-thirds of the hospitals in the United Kingdom and western Europe employ leeches for medicinal purposes, and the demand continues to rise. (Biopharm was even contacted during the notorious John Bobbitt incident, although the patient managed to heal without the aid of his slimy cousins.) The company sells fifty thousand leeches a year to hospitals and research labs in over twenty countries. Biopharm also maintains its own research program, and has isolated nearly fifty compounds with medical potential from just two species: the common European leech and the giant Amazon species. Ten of these natural compounds are so promising that they have been patented.

Once again, nature provides us with an invaluable service that we could not even have conceived of needing just a few decades ago. Who would have foreseen the reattachment of digits and limbs, much less predicted that it would have become an everyday, almost mundane practice? Surgeons now consider leeches indispensable for many microsurgical reattachments. And how long might it be before a scientist can design and build a contraption that can suck out excess blood, inject anticoagulants, attach itself to anywhere on the human body, and carry out all these tasks painlessly and inexpensively?

A sterling example that in many ways parallels the "rediscovery" of leeches is the use of maggots for the treatment of bone infections and other deep wounds. Western interest in maggot therapy has waxed and waned for the past 150 years, yet this treatment is known to have been a standard part of health-care practices among the Ngemba Aborigines of Australia, hill tribes of northern Burma, and Mayan healers in northern Central America. Ironically, many of the early observations of maggot therapy were made on the battlefields. Military surgeons like Baron Larrey of Napoleon's army noted that wounded soldiers who had lain abandoned on the battle-field and whose wounds were alive with wriggling maggots often healed better than those that received more immediate medical at-tention. Similar observations were made during the American Civil War and the First World War.

The "secret" of this peculiar medical practice is that the mag-gots of certain species of blowflies consume only putrefying tissues while, at the same time, they promote healing. The leading author-ity on maggot therapy is Dr. Ronald Sherman, a soft-spoken sur-geon at the University of California–Irvine School of Medicine who was originally trained as an entomologist. According to "The Maggot Man," as Dr. Sherman was christened when he appeared on the popular radio show *The People's Pharmacy*, these creatures help heal otherwise untreatable wounds by an amazing series of ac-tions: maggots eat and digest harmful bacteria, thus removing a major source of infection; they secrete therapeutic compounds like allantoin, ammonia, and calcium carbonate that sterilize the tis-sues; and they promote the growth of healthy tissue ("granulation tissue") by stimulation massage as they crawl through the wound. In many cases, wounds heal without the use of anesthesia or an-tibiotics, and leave fewer scars than those treated by traditional (and invasive) surgery.

Sherman says another advantage of what he has termed MDT (maggot debridement therapy) over surgery is that, unlike what sometimes happens when using surgical sponges, he doesn't have to worry about "leaving one in the patient." If a maggot dies in the wound during the course of therapy, the other maggots simply devour it. And eventually the maggots metamorphose into blow-flies, and fly away!

Maggot therapy has generated superb results in the treatment of osteomyelitis. This infection of the bone can occur after a break (like a compound fracture) exposes the internal tissues to germs, or as a result of an infection originating elsewhere in the body. Be-cause there is little blood circulation within the bone, once an in-fection is established, it is difficult for the body's immune system (or antibiotics in the blood system) to attack and defeat it. Without maggot therapy, the standard treatment is surgical removal of the infected area.

The use of maggots in modern medicine was first championed in this country over half a century ago by orthopedic surgeon Dr. William Baer of Johns Hopkins University. Hundreds of hospitals used maggots until the mid-1940s, when the practice was superseded by the widespread use of antibiotics and novel surgical techniques. However, according to Dr. Sherman, clinical studies by his research team are demonstrating that maggot therapy is more efficient at debriding (cleaning) infected and gangrenous wounds than any other nonsurgical treatment prescribed by the hospital's wound care team. "Wounds treated with MDT," he said, "healed many times more quickly than they had been healing prior to initiating MDT."

Furthermore, a 1932 report noted a different approach to using maggots medicinally: pulverizing them and placing the resulting mush directly into the wound. Some patients suffering from osteomyelitis and chronic leg ulcers were also vaccinated with the maggot mix. The success of this treatment implies that there may be more to maggot therapy than just consumption of diseased flesh. Indeed, maggots secrete three substances (allantoin and two others) that retard the growth of bacteria. And Sherman believes there are additional antibiotic compounds and has launched a project to find and isolate them.

Much of the recent search for new anticoagulants has focused on leeches and on snakes (as we'll see in the next chapter), but one intriguing lead has come from a totally unexpected source: the bark of a rain forest tree used as an arrow poison by an isolated tribe in the western Brazilian Amazon. Although the term *curare* is usually associated with arrow poisons employed by South American Indians, cultures around the world have employed toxic substances on the tips of their spears, darts, and arrows to make them even deadlier. In Homer's *Odyssey*, Ulysses seeks "the deadly poison wherewith to anoint his bronze-tipped arrows." So intertwined is the history of poison with that of the bow and arrow that the organic chemist John Mann noted the ancient Greek word *toxicon* (from which we derive toxic, toxin, toxicology, etc.) originally meant "poison for arrows."

Arrow poisons are and were most commonly used for hunting game, but they have been employed to kill everything from whales (by the Inuit people of the Arctic Circle), to wolves (in medieval Europe), to people. The South American curares were a source of great terror to the early explorers of the New World: the poison arrow was the only weapon that the Native Americans had that struck fear into the heart of the Spanish and English invaders. Unlike the blunderbuss (the firearm the invaders brought), it could be shot silently in the direction of the intended victim, and there was no antidote. Arrow poisons prepared from extracts of certain wild rubber trees caused a particularly excruciating death. Sir Walter Raleigh recorded what transpired: "The party shot indureth the most insufferable torment . . . and abideth a most ugly and lamentable death, sometimes dying stark mad, and in their frenzy biting their own hands and flesh from the extreme pain."

Amazonian curares cause relatively little pain, leading some historians to cast doubt on the veracity of accounts like Raleigh's. But one tropical American species of the rubber family can cause blinding pain, both by sensory nerve stimulation and by lowering the pain threshold.

The most common curares in South America are the moonseed species in the west and the strychnine species in the east. These plants contain alkaloids that interfere with the transmission of electrical impulses from the nerves to the muscles. Unable to receive signals from the nerves that usually control them, the muscles simply relax. One set of these muscles is the diaphragm, responsible for drawing air into the lungs. When the diaphragm relaxes to the point that it fails to function, the curarized person suffocates. Compounds derived from both the moonseed and the strychnine curares are employed in everything from open-heart surgery to rectal surgeries because physicians are able to use less of the (more dangerous) general anesthetic to relax the patient's skeletomuscular system. Interestingly, many of the original curare recipes prepared by the Indians included all or parts of venomous creatures like spiders, scorpions, ants, and snakes. The reductionist approach taken by Western scientists led to the testing of the "pure" plant extracts without the admixtures that may well augment the toxic (and possibly therapeutic) effect of the curare. Given the newfound interest in natural poisons by the pharmaceutical companies, the testing of both admixtures and newly discovered curares will undoubtedly become a priority in the not too distant future.

One novel curare from South America was brought to the attention of the outside world in the late 1980s. While attending meetings in Washington, D.C., about ten years ago, I received a phone call from *National Geographic* headquarters. The fellow on the other end of the line said that one of their Brazilian photographers was visiting and had brought back an interesting find that he wanted to discuss with "someone who knew something about arrow poisons of the Amazon." I walked over to their building and was met by a tall white-haired gentleman with a red face and a pronounced limp. As we shook hands, he introduced himself in English and Portuguese, both spoken with a thick German accent. "I'm Jesco von Puttkamer from Brazil," he said. "I have an arrow poison to show you. Follow me!"

I followed the old man into a brightly lit office at the end of the corridor. In the middle of the room was a light table covered with photographic slides. Expecting him to show me a picture, I was surprised when he reached over to a desk against the wall and picked up a dried leaf. "This is it!" he said, as if he had just handed me the answer to a riddle.

He explained that a recently contacted tribe of Indians called the Urueu-Wau-Wau in the remote jungles of western Brazil used this plant to make their curare. "I've been taking pictures in the Amazon for many decades now and this is unlike any arrow poison I've ever seen before," he explained. "First of all, these Indians make the poison from a tree but every other tribe I've lived with manufacture their curares from vines. Secondly, the wounds caused by arrows dipped in this curare cause the animals to bleed to death. What do you think it could be?"

The Amazon Basin harbors eighty thousand species of flowering plants. The leaves of many species are indistinguishable from one another. Moreover, the Western scientific system of plant classification is based on differences between the floral structures of plants. In other words, most botanists need to look at the flower— essentially the genitalia—to be able to identify the species. Giving a botanist a leaf from the Amazon and asking him or her to identify the species is akin to handing someone a car key and asking that person to describe the shape and color of the automobile it fits. One thing was certain: the leaf did not match up with the well-known species of either moonseed or strychnine curares, both of which feature distinctive leaves easily recognized by botanists.

Jesco was sufficiently familiar with curares to realize that he had stumbled across a new find. He returned to Urueu-Wau-Wau country, where he managed to collect more of the plant, including the bark from which the actual curare is prepared. The bark was sent to the New Jersey laboratories of Merck Pharmaceuticals, while the rest went to the New York Botanical Garden. At Merck, chemists found a new and potent anticoagulant from the bark and the sap of this plant. The plant extract inhibits both factor Xa and thrombin, thus interfering with the clotting cascade earlier than thrombin—in other words, it interferes with the clotting process in a unique manner, different than that of leech saliva or vampire bat saliva. Unfortunately, the plant molecule responsible for this effect turned out to be too toxic for medical use. Of course, technological tools often give us the ability to manipulate poisons so as to produce a therapeutic compound, as we saw with the cone snails.

Perhaps at least as intriguing as the chemical investigation was the botanical analysis at the New York Botanical Garden. There, Dr. Scott Mori, one of the toughest and most knowledgeable experts on the Amazonian flora, identified the species as *Cariniana domestica*, a tree of the Brazil nut tree family. In South America, this family is highly valued as a source of Brazil nuts and a bark that the Indians peel and use as straps for their backpacks. But, until the "discovery" of this obscure arrow poison, no one thought of this family as a source of powerful chemicals, much less a potent anticoagulant.

Leeches, vampire bats, and blowfly maggots offer little public appeal—in fact, most of us consider these species as downright loathsome. If these hideous healers can help us, imagine what other natural treasures still await discovery!

Chapter Six

THE SNAKES IN THE CADUCEUS

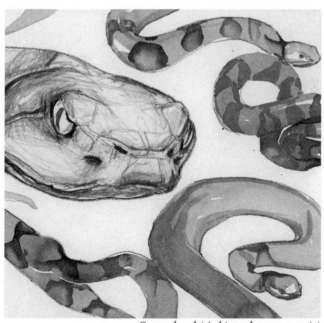

Copperhead (*Agkistrodon contortrix*)

What's wrong with snake oil? It works for me!
—Nigerian traditional Ibo healer

Eye of newt and toe of frog . . .
—The witches, in Shakespeare's *Macbeth*

The Andes comprise one of the world's longest and most rugged chains of mountains. Beginning at the southernmost tip of South America, just a few tens of miles off the coast of Antarctica, they run north for more than a hemisphere before gently petering out near the sandy shores of the Caribbean. Near the equator, the eastern escarpment plunges down into the great green depths of the Amazon rain forest. Snowcapped peaks stand sentinel over the hottest, wettest, most fecund forest on earth. Between these two extremes of temperature and altitude is a wild riot of microclimates in which almost every valley, almost every bend in the river holds some unique biological marvel. The American herpetologist Dr. William Duellman found as many frogs in this region as occur in all of the United States; the late lamented tropical botanist Dr. Al Gentry counted more species of trees in a single acre in this region than can be found on a similar sized plot of land anywhere else on the planet. And when the veteran South American explorer Loren McIntyre ventured there in October 1969, he witnessed something so peculiar, he worried that no one would believe it.

McIntyre fought in the Pacific during World War II. In the midst of the carnage that surrounded him, McIntyre made himself a promise: if he survived the war, he would devote his life to pursuing his childhood dream of exploring the Amazon. At the end of the war, he parlayed his military background into a posting in Peru.

Inspired by awesome scenery each time he left the dreary capital city of Lima, McIntyre worked hard at developing world-class photographic skills. His proficiency with the camera and his willingness to undertake the most challenging assignments quickly earned him a reputation as one of *National Geographic's* most accomplished photojournalists. He traveled the length and breadth of South America from the parched deserts of Santa Marta in the north to the frozen heights of Aconcagua in the south, living and traveling with tribes who had seen few outsiders. In the course of his rambles, McIntyre actually discovered the source lake of the Amazon, named Laguna McIntyre in his honor. Now in his early eighties, the wiry and weather-beaten McIntyre has lived a long and fascinating life. Still, no experience he ever had proved more unusual than what he witnessed deep in the jungles of the northwest Amazon in 1969.

Born in the Cordillera Ultra-Occidental in northern Peru, the Javari River flows in a northeast arc, first forming the Brazil-Peru border before emptying into the main body of the Amazon River just above the Colombian port town of Leticia. In October 1969, McIntyre hired a tiny single-engine Cessna floatplane to drop him near the headwaters of the Javari. Being alone and (for all intents and purposes) defenseless would, he hoped, help him make contact with the mysterious Mayoruna tribe. He had heard that these Indians wore "whiskers" made by inserting jungle grasses into their perforated nostrils in homage to the jaguar, which, as the most powerful and feared animal in the jungle, was sacred to their tribe.

The little plane landed and McIntyre unloaded his equipment onto a small sandy beach at the river's edge. The plane departed, and McIntyre busied himself by setting up camp. Before long, he felt several sets of eyes staring at him and managed to appear relaxed when several Indians wearing jaguarlike whiskers stepped out of the jungle. McIntyre spoke no Mayoruna and the Indians understood no Spanish or Portuguese. Using sign language, the Mayoruna invited the American to follow them into the forest, an invitation he readily accepted. As they hiked deeper into the forest, McIntyre began to question the wisdom of his decision when he and his newfound colleagues passed an abandoned Brazilian gold-mining site. The rotting skeletons of the miners looked like porcupines, so filled were they with Mayoruna arrows.

The Indians led McIntyre to a small encampment, where he spent a sleepless night in a Mayoruna palm thatch hut. The next morning all the warriors in the village lined up to dance, McIntyre among them. The slow, dirgelike music lasted for hours, and, at the end, everyone was painted with red *achiote* paste and blue *genipa* dye. A bowl of cassava beer was passed from hand to hand and McIntyre took a sip to quench his burning thirst. As he drank the sour potion, he watched several men open small arrowroot fiber baskets and pull out iridescent green monkey frogs with bulbous red-orange eyes.

In his book *Amazon Beaming*, Petru Popescu chronicled McIntyre's expedition and recorded what happened when the frogs came out of the baskets: "[The Indian] raises a knife of chonta palm and I turn away so as not to see him slice a frog but when I turn back I find him pulling the hard, sharp blade of wood away from his forearm and letting blood seep out of his torn skin. Immediately, two other [Indians] rush to take hold of his arm; they pull aside the lips of the bleeding wound, and pour liquid from a bowl of frog secretion into it. Straight into the bloodstream, for a quicker and more lasting effect."

Fifteen years later explorer-journalist Peter Gorman was traveling near where McIntyre had witnessed this strange ritual. An elderly Mayoruna shaman lay peacefully in his hammock as Gorman plied him with questions about indigenous use of plants and animals. Gorman pointed to a small bag of palm leaves that had been hung over a cooking fire to dry. At this, the shaman smiled and said one word: *sapo*, Spanish for toad.

The shaman climbed out of his hammock and untied the bag from over the fire. Unwrapping the bundle, he pulled out a small flat stick, one end of which was coated by a thick clear yellowish resin. He applied a dab of the compound to his left palm, spit into it, and rubbed it into a mustardlike paste with his right forefinger. Gorman watched transfixed as the shaman reached into the cooking fire and pulled out a smoldering twig. Before the American knew what was happening, the old Indian had grabbed Gorman's left wrist and burned two tiny holes on the inside of his left forearm. Gorman tried to pull away in surprise and pain, but the old man held fast. With the nail on his index finger, the shaman gently scraped the twin burns on the visitor's arm. Then he dabbed a little of the frog paste on the wounds. Thinking he was being shown the local treatment for burns, Gorman relaxed—but he shouldn't have: he was in for the ride of his life.

His body temperature skyrocketed as he felt himself burning from the inside out. Gorman's blood pressure shot up higher than it had ever been. His stomach collapsed in a gut-wrenching spasm, forcing him to vomit violently. Losing control of all of his bodily functions, he collapsed on the dirt floor in a heap.

"Suddenly, you may feel urges to do things you've never done before," wrote Gorman.

> You might find yourself growling, barking, or moving about on all fours. You feel as though animals are passing through you, trying to express themselves through your body. But even this extraordinary feeling is secondary to the speeding of your blood, a motion so fast you think your heart will burst. . . . The pain becomes so great that you wish you could die and get it over with but you don't die. . . . Finally the pounding subsides and you're overcome with exhaustion. You sleep. . . . There are no dreams or visions with *sapo*; you may even wonder what it was all for, until you wake—then you are a god! Everything about you is larger than life, and your physical strength is explosive. You can do without food for several days and run in the jungle for hours without tiring. You can see in the dark effortlessly. You see animals before they see you, and you sense which plants are benevolent and which are not. Every sense you possess is heightened and somehow in tune with the jungle, as though the *sapo* put the rhythm of the jungle in your veins.

Collections of *sapo* were sent to the National Institutes of Health in Bethesda, Maryland, by both Gorman and University of California anthropologist Dr. Katy Milton, who had observed similar rituals among Indian tribes in adjacent Brazil. They landed in the lab of Dr. John Daly, the godfather of frog chemistry who deciphered at least some of the mystery of other Amazonian amphibians. Daly passed some on to Dr. Vittorio Erspamer at the Fidia Research Institute for the Neurosciences in Rome. The results were almost as mind-blowing as Gorman's experience.

The *sapo* resin proved chock full of peptides, at least seven of which are highly bioactive, meaning they caused a specific reaction in the human body. Two of these peptides—caerulein and phyllocaerulein—have a strong effect on the gastrointestinal tract, increasing gastric and pancreatic secretions. These compounds cause nausea, vomiting, heart palpitations, sweating, and, most importantly, changes in blood pressure. And then there is the issue of pain: according to Erspamer, caerulein produces "an analgesic effect . . . possibly related to release of beta-endorphins . . . in patients suffering from renal colic, rest pain due to [limited circulation], and even cancer pain . . . [and] it caused a significant reduction in hunger and food intake." Caerulein is already being used experimentally in both Italy and Germany to lower blood pressure.

A frog-derived peptide named phyllomedusin affects the bowel and was probably the cause of the strong purge experienced by Gorman. Phyllokinin, another peptide found in the mixture, proved a highly effective blood vessel dilator and is therefore believed to be the cause of the intense "rush" that Gorman felt at the onset of the experience.

So impressed was Erspamer with the effectiveness of phyllomedusin and phyllokinin as vasodilators that he suggested that they may increase the permeability of the blood-brain barrier, another of the Holy Grails of modern medicine. Getting medicines from the blood into the brain is notoriously difficult—having the ability to do so may revolutionize treatments for debilitating diseases as AIDS, Alzheimer's, and certain cancers.

. . .

Due northwest of where McIntyre met the jaguar Indians and Gorman entered a godlike state, lies a land even less well known than the Amazon forest. This is the Choco, the western coastal strip of Colombia, which is one of the wettest places on earth. When Balboa stood atop the mountain in Darien and saw the Pacific Ocean stretching westward, his colleagues determined to sail south in search of riches that might equal those that de Soto had plundered from the Aztecs just a few years before. However, they were unable to get a foothold in western Colombia—every time they tried to land, clouds of poison-tipped arrows rained down upon them. Forced to continue sailing south, they eventually reached the land of the Inca nation. Unlike the curare-tipped darts of the Amazon, however, it is highly likely that the arrow's poison in the Choco was made not from plants, but from frogs.

In 1824, Captain Charles Cochrane of the British navy traveled through the steaming forests of the Choco. Despite a bout of malaria that nearly killed him, he managed to record the first account of an arrow poison extracted from a frog:

> Those who use this poison catch the frogs in the woods, and confine them in a hollow cane, where they regularly feed them until they want the poison, when they take one of the unfortunate reptiles [sic], and pass a pointed piece of wood down his throat, and out at one of his legs. This torture makes the frog perspire very much, especially on his back, which becomes covered with white froth: this is the most powerful poison that he yields, and in this they dip or roll the points of their arrows, which will preserve their destructive power for a year. . . . From one frog sufficient poison is obtained for about fifty arrows.

Biochemist John Daly's first encounter with this extraordinary creature twenty-five years ago left such an indelible impression that he remembers it as if it were yesterday. Biologist Boris Malkin had sent word to the United States that he had collected a new species of highly poisonous dart frog. He mailed it to amphibian expert Dr. Charles Myers at the American Museum of Natural History in New York, and Myers invited Daly up from Washington to have a look. The frogs proved so noxious that, as soon as Myers opened the container, a toxic cloud wafted out. The scientists' noses went numb and both began to sneeze uncontrollably. When they journeyed down to the Choco two years later, Daly prepared himself for working with the little amphibians by donning gloves, goggles, and a face mask. Even his proved insufficient: every night he'd go to bed with mucus gushing from his irritated nasal passages and half his face completely numb.

Daly and Myers observed the local Embera Indians extracting dart poison from frogs just as Cochrane had reported. The Indians are so fearful of the poison, however, that they refuse to handle the frogs directly, wrapping the tiny amphibians in leaves to pick them up, in sharp contrast to the plant-derived curares of Amazonia that the Indians handle with impunity.

Subsequent laboratory analysis in the United States quantified the astounding toxicity of the frog skin: 250 times more poisonous than Amazonian curare! Daly and his colleagues at the National Institutes of Health then began to break the poison down into separate components, not only to decipher what types of molecules were in the toxin, but to investigate whether these chemicals might prove beneficial for our own species.

The scientists encountered a plethora of new and potent compounds in the frog skin. So complicated are these chemicals that the name of one of them—isohydrohistrionicotoxin—is twice as long as the frog from which it is extracted! Another component, named batrachotoxin, has a powerful effect on sodium channels in the nervous system. By manipulating these channels with batrachotoxin from this rain forest frog, scientists have a better understanding of the function of local anesthetics, anticonvulsants, antiarrhythmics, and certain toxins.

Another class of compounds derived from these frogs—the pumiliotoxins—offers even greater promise. Pumiliotoxin exerts a cardiotonic action on the heart, similar to that of digitalis. The difference is that digitalis blocks an enzyme called sodium potassium

ATPase, which increases the rate and force of the heartbeat. Pumil-iotoxin works by delaying the opening and closing of the sodium channels, the tiny doorways on the surface of cells that control the amount of sodium that enters and departs. Consequently, every impulse that goes through the heart brings in more sodium, which in turn ushers in more calcium, which triggers a stronger contraction. Because it utilizes a different mechanism than digitalis to achieve the same end, pumiliotoxin (or a synthetic derivative) may one day prove useful in cases where digitalis is ineffective. Scientists are hoping that pumiliotoxin (or some derivative thereof) might one day be used to jump-start a heart that has been stilled by a heart attack.

Daly's work with the Colombian amphibians unleashed a wave of interest in novel compounds from frogs, particularly the psyche-delically colored members of the dart frog family. He and his colleagues have already discovered more than four hundred new chemicals in more than fifty species of these creatures, and no end is yet in sight. Medicinal applications are not restricted to compounds derived from dart frogs: Daly isolated a growth hormone in the European fire-bellied toad later found in human lung tumors. Physicians now test patients for this substance to determine whether lung tumors are present.

The most grotesque frog with potent chemicals in its skin is the *cururu,* the giant Amazon toad, which may reach a length of over a foot. The *cururu* (or "marine toad," as it has come to be known in the Western press for some unfathomable reason) is a lovely cream color which, combined with its huge size and grotesque shape, gives it a striking resemblance to Jabba the Hutt. The resemblance to the fictional *Star Wars* monster is heightened by its inclination to devour not only enormous quantities of insects but rodents, small reptiles, and even other frogs (!) that cross its path. Like many toads, this South American species harbors behind its eyes what are known as parotoid glands. These swollen glands are jam-packed with powerful chemicals both toxic and hallucinogenic. Dogs are often intrigued by these huge amphibians and bite them as an expression of curiosity. In this case, curiosity kills the dog rather than the cat.

Prevalent in the *cururu* is 5-hydroxy-N, N-dimethyltrypta-mine, a hallucinogenic compound common in many of the psy-choactive brews and snuffs prepared by Amazonian Indians from local plants. (Huge numbers of marine toad skeletons have been found in many Mayan ruins, leading some to hypothesize that these creatures played a role in pre-Columbian religious rites. Oth-ers have rebutted this argument, noting that larger specimens can be eaten if the poison glands are removed.)

Though the scientific evidence that Amazonian peoples have used these toads for healing purposes is, at best, inconclusive, tales of toad-licking as a means to experience other realities have been circulating in counterculture literature for at least thirty years. The experimentation with the *cururu*, however, has often produced dire results. In one instance, several people prepared soup from the frog's eggs (as we saw with the insects, species often deposit toxic substances in and around their eggs to deter predation). The results were fatal.

Of all the reptiles and amphibians—frogs, salamanders, newts, tu-ataras, crocodilians, turtles, and snakes—frogs and snakes offer the greatest promise as sources of new therapeutics. Lacking the shells of turtles or the teeth of crocodilians to defend themselves, frogs protect themselves with a passive defense: a plethora of powerful chemicals. But their reptilian cousins the snakes have also evolved a potent set of compounds that they employ for both offensive and defensive purposes.

Snakes have long served as objects of fascination and/or dread to many human cultures. From the serpent in the Garden of Eden in Judeo-Christian religions, to the giant anaconda that pulls the canoe of life in Tukanoan Indian tradition, snakes represent power, magic, knowledge, sex, death, and medicine. A creature without arms and legs that not only thrives but can kill a human with a sin-gle bite is a creature to be respected, feared, worshiped, and avoided, which is why Tutankhamen's death mask was crowned with a co-bra, and why one of colonial America's first flags featured a rat-tlesnake with the warning "Don't Tread on Me!" Poisonous snakes have served as agents of capital punishment, murder, suicide, torture, and even warfare (the Carthaginian general Hannibal won a naval engagement with the Romans by having his men toss pots filled with venomous serpents onto the enemy ship).

The association of snakes and healing also dates back thousands of years. Asclepius, Greek god of medicine, was believed to transform himself into a snake to cure people. His staff was an olive branch encircled by a snake. Known as the caduceus, this scepter serves as the symbol of modern medicine. Asclepius's temple at Epidaurus was inhabited both by rat snakes and priests of his cult, who proved to be skilled diagnosticians and dispensers of plant remedies as well. Sick people from all over the Mediterranean would sleep in the temple in the belief that the god would come in the night and either give advice or heal the patient himself.

Asclepius was said to have been schooled in the healing arts by both his father Apollo and Chiron the centaur, who also served as Hercules' tutor. The connection between Asclepius, healing, and snakes may have hinged on the serpent's habit of shedding its skin, a phenomenon often associated with rebirth and renewal around the world. This explains why Asclepius's staff features a stick entwined with a single serpent (*not* with two serpents, which is the symbol of Hermes, the winged-footed messenger of the gods). So great were the reptiles' reputed healing powers that the Romans brought them from Greece to Rome long before they imported Greek physicians!

One of the most common associations of snakes with healing (or the lack thereof) is the term "snake oil," which has a distinctively negative connotation in American culture. Patent medicine vendors of the traveling shows proved exceedingly popular in late-nineteenth-century America. Untrained in the medical arts, these pitchmen sold a variety of "healing elixirs" supposedly based on Native American medicinal herbs. Many were probably harmless and/or ineffective, some were poisonous, and others (laced with opium) were addictive. A not uncommon ingredient was snake fat or oil, hence the name "snake oil salesman." Ironically, in parts of West Africa, snake fat is valued as a high-quality massage oil. In

Nigeria, Ibo healers commonly employ massages with cobra fat as an effective treatment for certain neuralgias.

But the most important therapeutic compound snakes produce also happens to be the deadliest: venom. Snake poison does not consist of one single toxic substance; rather, it is typically a deadly cocktail of various toxins that, in some instances, can attack almost every organ system in the human body. Venoms not only vary from species to species; even snakes of the same species from corners of their geographic range may have poisons that differ. Snake poisons were once divided into two basic categories: neurotoxic (attacking the nervous system), which were said to be characteristic of cobras and their relatives; and hemotoxic (attacking the circulatory system), said to be characteristic of rattlesnakes and their relatives. As analytic tools in the lab have improved and as more venoms have been studied, the false dichotomy has broken down. Snakes once placed in one category were found to have venom that belonged in the other category or possessed venoms with both hemotoxic and neurotoxic attributes.

Each species of poisonous snake possesses its own unique venom that often serves both as a toxin to immobilize and kill prey, and as a pool of enzymes to initiate the digestive process. Most of these poisons are effective and quick acting, desirable qualities of pharmaceuticals. And each of the toxic compounds has been exquisitely engineered through the evolutionary process to attack a specific part of the blood and/or nervous system.

The sheer variety of snake venom offers a cornucopia of compounds with enormous therapeutic potential. So great is this potential that the venoms of over eighty species of poisonous snakes, everything from the common cottonmouth moccasin of my home state of Louisiana to more exotic species like the African spitting cobra, are commercially available from chemistry supply houses for laboratory testing. Steve Grenard, a leading authority on the medical applications of reptiles and amphibians, notes that fractions obtained from snake venom have been used in the treatment and diagnosis of epilepsy, high cholesterol, pain, emphysema, osteoporosis, cancer, blood clotting abnormalities, HIV/AIDS, and high blood pressure. The last led to the development of one of the most lucrative drugs in the history of Western medicine.

High blood pressure is one of the most common causes of death in the human species, particularly in the industrialized world where a sedentary lifestyle and fat-rich diet prevail. On the African savannas, where our species first arose, our heart pumped overtime in fight-or-flight situations. This intensified blood flow through constricted arteries might provide the energy necessary to outrun a hungry lion, but will burn out an emotionally stressed human body continuously parked behind an office desk or in front of a computer monitor or television set. More than sixty million Americans suffer from this disease, termed "the silent killer" because countless people die not having known they were ill. Hypertension causes a particularly detrimental effect on the blood vessels of the brain, heart, and kidneys. Left untreated, high blood pressure often leads to heart attack, stroke, and kidney failure.

As recently as the 1960s, scientists were still having enormous difficulty deciphering the causes, and the potential treatments, for this syndrome. Some believed high blood pressure was the result of too much pumping of the blood by the heart muscle, while others postulated that it was due to the retention of an overabundance of water in the body. The third theory, later proven correct, was that the problem was primarily caused by constriction of the smooth muscles that make up much of the blood vessel walls.

During the 1960s, Brazilian scientists became curious as to why people bitten by the *jararacussu*, a six-foot-long, yellow-brown pit viper related to the rattlesnake and native to the grasslands of eastern Brazil, died not only in great pain, but also from a blood pressure level so low that it could be fatal in and of itself. While synthetic chemists in the United States created compound after compound in a fruitless attempt to develop a medicine to lower blood pressure, the Brazilians began to wonder if Mother Nature had already done so.

In the early 1960s, the Brazilian pharmacologist Dr. Mauricio Rocha e Silva at the University of São Paulo hypothesized that the pain and inflammation caused by the bite of the *jararacussu* resulted from the presence of histamine, a common component of animal venoms. He took some of the snake venom and injected it into a dog. He then drew blood from the dog and squirted it over a piece of human intestinal muscle, knowing that, in the presence of histamine, the muscle would quickly contract. Rocha e Silva tried this experiment several times, yet the muscle did not react. Disappointed, he went home.

His student Wilson Beraldo remained in the lab and, out of a mixture of both boredom and curiosity, tried again. Slowly, like a scene out of an old Frankenstein movie, the muscle came to life and began to move. Yet it was not the sharp, immediate contraction typically caused by histamine. Instead, it was a slow and steady response, caused by a different compound. The Brazilians christened this new chemical *bradykinin,* a term created by joining the Greek words for "slow" (*bradys*) and "to move" (*kinein*). Ironically, bradykinin doesn't exist in the venom itself, but is formed from compounds in the blood of the snakebite victim once it comes into contact with the reptile's poison. This is why the muscle didn't contract in Rocha's lab immediately after it was exposed to the poison—it took a while for the bradykinin to form and take effect.

Rocha learned that this substance caused two intriguing reactions when injected: it induced terrible pain and it lowered blood pressure. Wanting to learn more, scientists returned to the *jararacussu* venom. A research team led by the Brazilian Dr. Sergio Ferreira isolated a peptide that inhibits an enzyme that breaks down bradykinin. This find elucidated one of the nefarious ways that the venom works: it not only causes the release of a painful compound (bradykinin), it also produces another compound that prevents the conversion of angiotensin I to angiotensin II, which constricts the blood vessels, thereby raising blood pressure. A chemical that could inhibit the production of angiotensin-converting enzyme (in other words, an ACE inhibitor) should be able to lower blood pressure.

The scientists faced several major obstacles that had to be overcome if their research was to result in a new treatment for high blood pressure. A research team that included the American Dr. David Cushman and the Argentine Dr. Miguel Ondetti led an international effort to identify the peptide responsible for inhibiting angiotensin I to angiotensin II. Unfortunately, a gram of *jararacussu* venom contained only a millionth of a gram of the peptide. Capturing enough deadly pit vipers to extract a quantity of venom sufficient for the treatment of millions of patients in the United States alone was not only impractical but also immensely unappealing. Furthermore, peptides degrade in the human digestive system, so developing a pill containing the peptides was also unfeasible. Furthermore, people would be unlikely to self-administer injections of the peptide three times a day.

Inspired by the compound in the snake's poison known as teprotide, the scientists developed a synthetic compound that could be taken orally and would be an inhibitor of the action of the angiotensin-converting enzyme, thereby lowering blood pressure. The drug, known as captopril (Capoten), succeeded beyond their wildest dreams. It eventually became Bristol-Myers Squibb's most lucrative product, generating 1.66 billion dollars in 1992 alone. Not only was captopril found to be effective as a medicine for high blood pressure, but it lacked many of the side effects associated with other antihypertension drugs. Furthermore, captopril also proved highly effective in treating certain forms of congestive heart failure as well as slowing the progression of kidney disease in people suffering from diabetes. Steve Grenard said, "[Captopril] has saved the lives of millions of people, sparing them from death and disability due to stroke, cerebral hemorrhage, aneurysms, heart and kidney disease."

And subsequent research on this same venom by Ferreira and his colleagues has found additional compounds that may prove three times more effective than captopril.

New medicines continue to be developed from other snake venoms. We are finding additional ACE inhibitors (like enalapril) from other species. And these reptile poisons offer great hope for treating blood problems other than hypertension.

The venoms of several poisonous species contain both coagulants and anticoagulants, making treatment in these cases fiendishly difficult. These venoms, however, are of obvious interest to scientists, particularly those researchers engaged in the development of novel treatments for blood disorders. One of these venoms led directly to tirofiban (Aggrastat), a new anticoagulant that the pharmaceutical giant Merck recently brought to market.

Dr. Robert Gould, executive director of pharmacology at Merck, was interested in new treatments that could prevent heart attacks and other cardiac disorders. He knew that unstable angina, characterized by often severe chest pains, was perhaps the most common reason for emergency room admissions in the United States. Angina is caused by diminished blood flow to the heart muscle. If you can re-invigorate the blood supply to the heart, you can reverse unstable angina and prevent a potentially fatal heart attack in the future.

In fact, many (if not most) people have some narrowing of the coronary arteries (the precursor to both unstable angina and myocardial infarctions, better known as heart attacks) due to the presence of cholesterol and plaque. What kills you during a heart attack is not the diminished blood flow due to coronary occlusion, but the formation of a blood clot that closes off the artery completely, starving the heart of oxygen. If you can interfere with the formation of the clot, you should be able to prevent the attack.

Platelets, tiny components in the blood, play a key role in the coagulation cascade, as we saw in Chapter 5. They are, in Gould's words, "the first line of defense that keeps you from bleeding to death when you have a cut." The problem, though, was that the platelets would sometimes begin sticking to each other in already-clogged cardiac arteries, which could be fatal.

Gould and his colleagues knew that the bite of certain poisonous snakes caused victims to bleed to death. They hypothesized that these venoms might contain a compound capable of interfering with the coagulation cascade in a manner that could prevent heart attacks and other blood problems. In collaboration with colleagues at Temple University in Philadelphia, they purified and tested the venoms of many different species of poisonous snakes from around the world. They hit paydirt with the saw-scaled viper.

Found primarily in shrubby arid regions of Africa and Asia, the saw-scaled viper feeds on both lizards and rodents. This snake has a most peculiar habit: by rubbing together the ridges on its scales, it produces an unmistakable rasping sound dreaded in the Old World at least as much as the hissing of the rattlesnake in North America. The poison of the saw-scaled viper, however, tends to be infinitely more lethal. Though only two feet in length, the viper is both aggressive and irritable; its bite causes severe (and often fatal) hemorrhaging. The saw-scaled viper and its larger cousin, the Russell's viper, probably kill more people each year than any other two species of snakes. How ironic, then, that the deadly venom of the saw-scaled viper led to the development of a new drug that will save millions of lives.

Gould and his colleagues' goal was to find (or develop) a molecule that would interfere with platelets' ability to adhere to each other. Most cells in the body have the capability of sticking to other cells, so the object of Gould's quest had to be exquisitely selective in terms of what cells it impacted. He found a compound in the viper venom that blocked the platelets from adhering to each other, but it also had side effects in the human body. He and his colleagues at Merck then used the molecule from the snake poison as a model for a synthetic compound that lacked the deleterious effects on other cells. The new molecule, tirofiban, is in widespread use just a year after it was approved by the FDA. The drug is expected to reduce heart attacks and deaths by 50 percent among patients suffering from unstable angina. Merck estimates that tirofiban is already preventing forty thousand heart attacks and ten thousand fatalities a year. According to Gould, "without the knowledge [we gathered from studying] this snake venom, we would not have been able to design a small molecule which, when infused into patients, can prevent unstable angina, myocardial infarction, and death."

Unlike tirofiban, which is a synthetic product *based* on compounds found in snake venom, the anticoagulant ancrod (Arvin) occurs in nature. Scientists studying the survivors of Malayan pit-viper bites noticed that their blood was extremely thin and barely clotted. Each year, half a million Americans suffer strokes, 10 percent of which are fatal. Because more than 75 percent of all strokes are caused by blood clots, investigators hypothesized that this poison might harbor therapeutic potential. They were able to isolate the compound, which dissolves some clots and, by decreasing blood thickness, prevents the formation of others. As with many drugs, ancrod may also help to cure ailments other than the one it was developed to treat. Researchers believe that this snake venom compound offers hope for the treatment of acute ischemic stroke, caused by reduced blood flow to the brain. And other anticoagulants are being developed from domestic species like the southern copperhead and the western diamondback rattlesnake.

Moreover, these venom-derived drugs for blood disorders have inspired a promising new lead for the treatment of cancer. Snake venoms cause hemorrhages by interfering with integrin proteins on cell surfaces that play a vital role in clotting. Tirofiban functions as a disintegrin—it impedes the action of integrins. Dr. Francis Markland at the University of Southern California knew that integrins on tumor cells resemble those on blood platelets—so why not search for disintegrins that would keep cancer cells from aggregating?

Markland found what he was looking for in the venom of the copperhead, a gorgeous orange-brown viper of the southeastern United Sates. The disintegrin he isolated from the copperhead—named contortrostatin after the scientific name for the copperhead (*contortrix*)—kept the cancer cells from sticking to healthy tissue and prevented them from growing the blood vessels necessary to nourish themselves. Unlike many compounds used in chemotherapy, whose toxicity not only affects the cancer cell but sometimes negatively impacts healthy cells, contortrostatin puts tumors to sleep by choking off their ability to feed themselves and grow. Though research is still very preliminary—the drug has been tested only in mice and not yet in humans—the results are very promising: growth of breast cancer cells was reduced 70 percent, while spread of lung cancer cells was reduced 90 percent.

. . .

Despite increasing public awareness of the value of tirofiban, and potential new drugs like contortrostatin, many species of reptiles and amphibians face possible extinction. Amphibians represent probably the single most endangered group of vertebrates. Some of the most spectacular species of frogs are threatened by greedy and unscrupulous American and European collectors for the pet trade. Turtles and snakes are also overharvested for this commercial enterprise.

At least as grave a threat, and probably a more serious one, is that of habitat disturbance. The southern copperhead, source of contortrostatin, thrives in southern woodlands of the United States, which are being converted to housing developments. Once-pristine sea turtle nesting beaches are covered with resort hotels. But the group most heavily impacted by habitat conversion is the amphibians.

Amphibians were the first vertebrates to leave the oceans and colonize dry land. Most are still tied to the water at some stage of their life. They may inhabit terrestrial environments for most of their adult life, but the majority of species lay their eggs in water. With the global effort to drain the wetlands, either to provide yet more living space for an ever-increasing human population or to reduce the populations of malaria-infected mosquitoes, amphibian habitats and the amphibians themselves are declining every year. Their porous skin adds to their vulnerability. The many toxins we are forever pumping into the environment are readily absorbed by these creatures, reducing their ability to reproduce successfully or simply killing them outright.

And yet another human-caused environmental disruption is also having a devastating consequence: the greenhouse effect. A precipitous decline in frog populations was first noted around the world in the early 1990s. Scientists believe that the greenhouse effect, which has had such a deleterious effect on the ozone layer, is allowing gamma rays to penetrate the atmosphere and scramble the DNA in frog eggs, which seem particularly susceptible. Some have warned that we should consider amphibians to be the modern-day equivalents of the coal miner's canary, in that whatever is killing these small animals is having a less obvious but inexorable effect on us as well.

Perhaps the sad story of the Australian gastric brooding frog best exemplifies what can be lost when a single species disappears. In 1974, Australian herpetologist Dr. Michael Tyler of the University of Adelaide found a new species of frog living in boulder-strewn, fast-flowing rain forest creeks in the Canondale Range of Queensland. Unlike John Daly's brilliantly colored poison dart frogs, these amphibians were fairly nondescript, with brown backs and cream-colored undersides. But this species exhibited a peculiar behavior: the females swallowed their own eggs, incubated them in their stomachs, and gave birth through their mouths. A single frog hatched out twenty-one frogs in the same litter!

How was this amphibian—christened "the Australian gastric brooding frog"—able to carry the eggs (and then the tadpoles) inside her stomach without having everything digested by the stomach acid? The mother frog was found to have the ability to turn off her stomach acids while carrying both the eggs and the tadpoles.

"If we could have found out what turned off the frog's stomach acids and other gastric activity to permit it to gestate its eggs for six weeks," said Steve Grenard, "such a find could have translated into an important medical advance, especially in the treatment of gastric hyperacidity and human ulcer disease."

Unfortunately, we can't find out what turned off the frog's stomach acids or whether there was therapeutic potential for our own species—the Australian gastric brooding frog went extinct in 1980.

Chapter Seven

UNDER
THE SEA

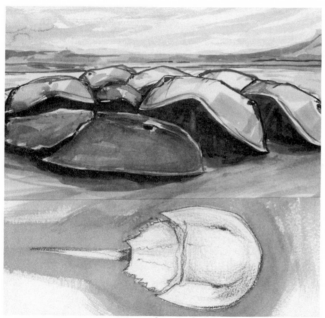

Horseshoe crab (*Limulus polyphemus*)

All that we do is touched with ocean,
yet we remain on the shore of what we know . . .
—Richard Wilbur, former U.S. poet laureate

Full fathom five thy father lies;
of his bones are coral made . . .
—Ariel, in Shakespeare's *The Tempest*

On a balmy December day off the northwest coast of Australia, Dr. William Fenical was not looking for new medicines from the sea when he strapped on his scuba tanks, dove into the ocean, ignored the sharks that kept lunging into him, and discovered one of the most potent anticancer compounds ever found.

Fenical, director of the Center for Marine Biotechnology at the prestigious Scripps Institution of Oceanography in San Diego, is Indiana Jones with an aqualung. He and his colleagues are at the forefront in exploring the planet's largest and least-known ecosystem: the ocean. With nets, scuba, sonar, and submarines both manned and unmanned, they are combing the seven seas in search of Mother Nature's most inaccessible healing magic.

Fenical's expedition was merely an exploratory visit to determine whether the area harbored new and unknown species. Ferried to Bennett's Shoal off the town of Exmouth by an ancient local guide with a sizable paunch and a few old bullet-wound scars in his chest, the American donned his tanks, flippers, and mask. As he placed the regulator in his mouth and prepared to enter the water, the Australian offered a last-minute piece of advice: "Careful, mate, the bloody place is crawlin' with big sharks!"

Having dived with sharks on many occasions, Fenical was cautious but unperturbed. What bothered him, however, as he entered the water and cleared his mask, was the unexpected murkiness. From the boat, he had estimated that the visibility would extend to thirty or forty feet, but the current had changed, and he could barely make out the gloves he wore. An optimist by nature, Fenical assumed that the murk would soon clear, and he'd then be able to search for unusual marine organisms. He had momentarily forgotten the skipper's warning when something big shoved him from behind. He turned, but was unable to see anything, so he decided it must have been the currents shifting. Then it happened again. And again.

Believing himself surrounded by aggressive sharks he could not see, the biologist considered ascending to the safety of the boat when the murk cleared in a manner reminiscent of DeMille's depiction of the Red Sea parting:

> In front of me were a series of boulders, about six feet high. On them were growing peculiar soft corals unlike any I had ever seen before. . . . They were shaped like human fingers, four or five inches long. . . . Some were bright red, while others were yellow. They were brightly colored and conspicuously positioned, but none of the fish or other creatures had taken any bites out of them, so I thought they must harbor some interesting chemicals. I collected a few, carried them up to the boat, put them in a plastic bag, placed them in an ice chest, had them shipped home and promptly forgot about them.

Many months later, a German scientist visiting from the University of Heidelberg entered Fenical's office, clearly excited. "What do you think about this?" he asked. On Fenical's desk he placed several sheets of paper, one of which featured the chemical structure of a new type of compound, along with data describing the substance's effectiveness at killing cancer cells in the test tube. Its efficacy, says Fenical, was "extremely whopping." The compound represented one of the most effective cancer-cell killers that

Fenical had ever seen. The American was elated. "Where did you get this compound?" he asked.

The German replied, "I was looking through your freezer and found these peculiar soft corals, so I cut off a small piece and ran this analysis. Isn't this great?"

Fenical was both excited and annoyed. Though he had obtained the permits necessary for collecting the organism, he hadn't planned on testing it medicinally, which required an additional set of permits from the Australian government. Obtaining this sort of "after the fact" permission is often fiendishly difficult, but the scientist knew he would have to persevere. Once all the paperwork had been completed, some of the world's top natural product chemists decided to synthesize the chemical, which they named eleutherobin. It took more than three years to produce this anticancer compound in the laboratory.

Cancer is not a single disease: more than a hundred different varieties exist. What characterizes all cancers is the uncontrolled growth of cells that assume abnormal shapes and cease normal function. Consequently, many of the most effective anticancer drugs selectively poison these abnormal cells (or at least prevent them from reproducing) with minimal harm to most normal cells. The alkaloids of the pink-flowered rosy periwinkle from Madagascar represent a classic example. Cells reproduce through a five-step process known as mitosis, where the chromosomes form a line, replicate, and are pulled apart by spindles into each half of the newly forming cell. The periwinkle alkaloids function as spindle poisons, destroying the spindles and thereby preventing the cancer cell from reproducing. Because they attack only the rapidly dividing cells, these compounds are more scalpels than sledgehammers.

Eleutherobin attacks cancer cells in a different manner. Like taxol, the ovarian cancer drug derived from the Pacific yew tree, it thwarts the cancer by binding to its microtubules, cellular structures that facilitate cell division. The microtubules become rigid and are unable to divide, thereby preventing the cancerous cell from reproducing. Though the means of attacking the cancer cell resembles that of taxol, the chemical structure bears little resemblance to the yew-derived compound. Fenical and his colleagues believe that eleutherobin may prove more effective than taxol at treating breast and ovarian cancer. If not, eleutherobin might be useful in treating taxol-resistant cancers.

One obstacle prevents the scientists from testing these hypotheses and possibly bringing this drug to market: the supply of eleutherobin. Harvesting every piece of the soft coral in the world capable of producing eleutherobin would not produce enough of the chemical to meet the demand for clinical testing. And, even though scientists have managed to synthesize the compound, the process they developed is still too expensive to yield a sufficient quantity of eleutherobin for testing purposes. Clinical development of a promising treatment for breast and ovarian cancer has come to a screeching halt because we cannot make eleutherobin as cheaply or effectively as a tiny soft coral off the coast of Australia.

Eleutherobin represents only one of the promising anticancer leads from the ocean. Marine organisms known as blue-green algae (though they are more closely related to bacteria than green algae) offer the same (or even greater) potential. They represent one of the most ancient of all living groups of organisms: having evolved almost three million years ago, they may well have been the source of much of the original oxygen in the primeval atmosphere. Blue-green algae (also known as cyanobacteria) often produce highly toxic compounds, the therapeutic potential of which is only now being realized. Because numerous species of blue-green algae produce toxic compounds, scientists like Fenical have long believed they offer great potential as anticancer drugs. This hypothesis has been proven correct with the discovery of blue-green-algae-derived compounds call cryptophycins, one of the most promising groups of natural chemicals ever found.

Scientists realized the power of these cryptophycins when several researchers contracted severe dermatitis after merely handling the algae. Research showed that these compounds not only have anticancer potential but exhibit antiviral effects as well—at least in the test tube—against RSV (respiratory syncytial virus, a common children's respiratory ailment), herpes, and even HIV.

Dr. Richard Moore and Dr. Susan Mooberry of the University of Hawaii have spearheaded the development of these new drugs that, like taxol and eleutherobin, destabilize cellular microtubules. A recent article in the prestigious *Journal of the American Medical Association* by researchers at Wayne State University School of Medicine discussed the use of cryptophycins to treat human breast and prostate cancer implanted in mice and found the results exceedingly promising.

Similar experiments with colon tumors were also successful. The scientists in Hawaii working on cryptophycins went on to claim that, in animal studies, these chemicals appear to be "superior to all commercially available clinical drugs tested in that they were also highly effective against drug-resistant tumors." This is particularly important for cases where tumor growth resumes after the cancer has become resistant to the drug being used, much the same as bacteria often develop resistance to antibiotics.

As was the case with eleutherobin, cryptophycins can be synthesized, but the cost of doing so is prohibitive. Unlike the case of eleutherobin, however, pharmaceutical giant Eli Lilly stepped in and is collaborating with the scientists to test and commercialize the drug. Using combinatorial chemistry, the researchers have developed more than two hundred different versions of the original molecule. Though bringing a new drug to the marketplace is an arduous and expensive process, Fenical feels that this is a drug that is "going places."

What makes the sea so promising a source of new pharmaceuticals? One obvious reason: the sheer volume of the aquatic domain, which covers over 70 percent of our planet. Some marine biologists have suggested that 80 percent of all species will eventually be found underwater. Whereas many terrestrial organisms (bacteria, mammals, etc.) have aquatic cousins, numerous groups of sea creatures (starfish/echinoderms, sponges/tunicates) have virtually no terrestrial counterparts, increasing the likelihood that they harbor unique chemical compounds. Of the approximately thirty-five different groups (phyla) of organisms that inhabit our planet, more than twenty dwell only underwater. Fenical has pointed out that a single drop of seawater may harbor eighty thousand microorganisms, most of which have never been studied.

Many researchers in drug development consider the ocean realm to be the most promising ecosystem for finding new medicines. The major pharmaceutical firms—Merck, Lilly, Pfizer, Hoffman-LaRoche, Bristol-Myers Squibb—have established marine biology divisions. At the same time, we are seeing an explosion of small companies like Cal Bio Marine, Oceanix Biosciences, and Pharma Mar whose major focus is new drugs from the sea. The first new ocean-derived pharmaceuticals to hit the market—which will happen in the next few years—will undoubtedly lead to an even greater stampede into these watery realms. But the historical precedent for aquatic medical research was set a half century ago, when a single species of aquatic microbe provided us with our most commonly used weapon against infectious disease.

Though penicillin proved to be a "miracle drug" for the treatment of many ailments when developed in the 1940s, it did not cure afflictions caused by gram-negative bacteria. Even if it had been widely available in 1945 (which, because of the war, it was not), the drug would not have been a panacea on the Mediterranean island of Sardinia, where typhoid (caused by gram-negative bacteria) rampaged. Italian chemist Dr. Giuseppe Brotzu, a microbiologist who served as chancellor of the University of Cagliari in Sardinia, devised an ingenious solution. To find an antibiotic effective against typhoid, he reasoned, he needed a microorganism that either fed on or was able to coexist with the bacilli that caused the disease. Since typhoid was a water-borne disease, he collected water samples where the storm drains of Cagliari emptied into the Mediterranean. Here, he hypothesized, he might find not only harmful bacteria, but also microorganisms capable of fending them off.

Brotzu's hunch proved correct. He found an aquatic mold, *Cephalosporium acremonium*, which led to the development of the cephalosporin antibiotics, currently the most commonly prescribed antibiotics in American hospitals. Cephalosporins destroy many gram-negative bacteria and some penicillin-resistant gram-positive bacteria, can be used in treating a wide variety of infections, and are relatively nontoxic. Pharmaceutical chemists have developed more than twenty derivatives with a range of different antibiotic activity and continue to create new versions. The current retail value of cephalosporin antibiotics exceeds one billion dollars per year.

Not all of the future drugs from the sea are being developed from microorganisms. The seas teem with little-known soft-bodied organisms. Like terrestrial plants, these shell-less organisms often deter their predators by chemical warfare. These marine creatures often teem with exquisitely potent poisons, the complexity and therapeutic potential of which we are only now beginning to appreciate and harness for our own purposes.

David Newman of the National Cancer Institute recently remarked, "If you are fat, fleshy, brightly colored and slow moving, I want to see you. There's something in you, on you, or traveling with you that stops you from being eaten." Or, more succinctly, the creature with the best chemistry set wins.

Emblematic of the mystery and potential are entire ecosystems at the bottom of the sea. Around hydrothermal vents on the ocean floor, where boiling hot water and toxic chemicals spew forth, live bizarre groupings of extraordinarily peculiar organisms. As seen in Chapter 2, creatures thriving in boiling water and consuming toxic chemicals are what led to the development of the polymerase chain reaction.

These bizarre microbes comprise just one tier of complete ecosystems found in an area that scientists once considered devoid of life. Since the first hydrothermal vents were discovered near the Galápagos in 1977, researchers have found giant tubeworms, hairy snails, blind crabs, and clams the size of dinner plates thriving in these nether realms. Who knows what else is out (or down) there?

The chemicals that we are finding in oceanic creatures are so new, so unlike anything encountered in terrestrial species, that they demonstrate activity against a panoply of ailments incurable with currently available medicines. Though still relatively ignorant of what exactly is to be found twenty thousand leagues under the sea, we have already identified antibiotics, anticancer agents, anti-inflammatories, and analgesic compounds. Cod liver oil has long served as an important (if repugnant) source of vitamins A and D. The hormone calcitonin, extracted from salmon, interferes with activity of specialized bone cells called osteoclasts, which absorb bone tissue; thereby calcitonin prevents osteoporosis. And protamine sulfate from salmon sperm (!) provides us with an antidote to the anticoagulant heparin. Even extinct species play a role: the antiseptic ichthammol is made from coals formed from the bodies of fossilized fishes!

Until recently, several factors proved almost insurmountable barriers to the development of new drugs from the sea. The most basic: we are terrestrial organisms. Not until the development of scuba by Jacques Cousteau and his colleagues after World War II were we able to penetrate deep water on a regular basis. And even scuba has severe limitations: divers using the apparatus are, for the most part, operating at a maximum depth of 120 feet, meaning that the vast majority of the ocean is out of bounds. And "the deep" takes on new meaning when applied to the ocean: if you took Mount Everest, at 28,000 feet the highest point on earth, and placed it in the Marianas Trench (the deepest part of the ocean), the mountain's summit would still be a mile below the ocean's surface! Even the so-called midwaters, halfway to the ocean floor, teem with life, contrary to what many oceanographers long believed. The midwater is home to the giant squid, a genuine sea monster that has fired the imagination of writers, biologists, and seafarers since our species first sailed into the open ocean. Exceeding sixty feet in length, these titanic mollusks may weigh over half a ton. More than half a century since splitting the atom, more than thirty years since landing a man on the moon, and over a decade after finding and photographing the wreck of the *Titanic*, we still have not been able to find, capture, and study a living specimen of the giant squid.

Another challenge of the sea exemplified by Fenical's work with eleutherobin: obtaining sufficient specimen quantities for laboratory testing and clinical evaluation. The anticancer compound ecteinascidin, from a Caribbean sea squirt, offers promise as a treat-

ment for melanoma and breast cancer. But a ton of these tiny creatures yields only a gram of the compound. One investigator began
research on marine microorganisms forty years ago and needed to
grow two thousand liters of the microbe to extract ten milligrams
of the protein being studied. With superior technology and growing techniques available, what once took him more than a year can
be accomplished today in less than two weeks.

Our ever improving technology continues to facilitate our ability to find, study, and utilize marine organisms for a multitude of
purposes. And no sea creature better symbolizes how a "primitive"
creature can provide us with important medicinal compounds than
the lowly sponge. This seemingly mundane invertebrate is proving
to be a biochemical titan. While many historians have written of
the ancient relationship between humans and dogs, we have probably been using sponges almost as long as we have shared our
dwellings with canines. The ancient Greeks dove for sponges, which
have been employed for thousands of years as everything from
mops to paint brushes to drinking vessels. During the Middle Ages,
burnt sponges were employed for medicinal purposes. And no
modern operating room would be complete without an ample supply of surgical sponges.

Although a few species do exist in fresh water, most sponges
prefer warm marine environments. In a sense, they represent the
marine equivalent of terrestrial plants: they cannot flee from
predators, so they dissuade them by other (usually chemical)
means. Sponges vary greatly in size, from a quarter inch to over
several yards. By virtue of the fact that some species have simple
digestive and circulatory systems, sponges are considered animals
even though they lack true tissues or organs. They have proven extraordinarily adept at developing mutually beneficial relationships
with everything from crustaceans to microorganisms. *Dromia*
crabs camouflage themselves by planting a sponge on the back of
their shells, while hermit crabs sometimes carry a sponge around
with them. Certain species of shrimps, corals, starfish, mollusks,
fish, brown algae, blue-green algae, and even a Christmas-like as-
sortment of both red and green algae live in or around particular

sponges, protected by the disagreeable taste and odor of these primitive creatures.

Yet we are finding that it is often not the sponges themselves that produce these unpleasant (and often medicinally intriguing) substances. Rather, the microscopic organisms living in or on the sponges are responsible. So complex are these relationships that some researchers have called sponges more of a living consortium than a single creature. The tiny creatures that comprise much of the sponge's defense system are reminiscent of Augustus De Morgan's nineteenth-century quote on biodiversity:

> Great fleas have little fleas upon their backs to bite 'em
> And little fleas have lesser fleas and so ad infinitum!

While scientists are busy deciphering which of these novel therapeutic agents are produced by the sponges themselves and which are manufactured by their microscopic partners, one thing is for certain: the study of sponges has already provided us with some of the most important drugs ever discovered.

Shortly after the Second World War, the Swedish biochemist W. Bergmann began studying the *Cryptotheca crypta* sponge of the Florida Keys. He brought specimens to his lab at Yale and began the analysis. After adding a solvent to the flask, he noticed a white substance forming that piqued his curiosity. Further investigation revealed that the compound represented a new type of nucleoside (nucleosides are the basic building blocks of DNA and RNA). Bergmann and his colleagues eventually isolated two novel biologically active nucleosides, which he called spongouridine and spongithymidine. He published the results in 1955.

Less than a decade later, others were inspired by Bergmann's discoveries to synthesize novel chemicals based on the structure of these sponge-derived chemicals. One of these compounds, cytosine arabinoside (also known as ara-C), quickly proved to be an effective treatment for leukemia and entered the marketplace in 1969. Thirty years later, ara-C remains one of our most effective treatments for this dreaded disease.

French chemists studying the anticancer efficacy of Bergmann's sponge made a startling observation: it also killed certain viruses. This was, in one sense at least, even more exciting than finding a new treatment for cancer. Viruses are tiny, tiny intracellular parasites consisting of a piece of DNA or RNA wrapped in a protective coat, usually of protein. They cause a wide range of human diseases, ranging from annoyances like chicken pox and warts to more lethal ailments like rabies and AIDS. They tend to function by hijacking a normal cell and forcing it to do their bidding, such as producing copies of the virus itself since the virus cannot reproduce on its own.

Even today, there are very few medicines that can successfully treat a virus without harming the cell that the virus has invaded. The scientists who observed the antiviral capability of this Caribbean sponge quickly synthesized a related compound. Known as adenine arabinoside, vidarabine, or ara-A, it is used against both herpes and shingles. Ara-A was the first safe and effective antiviral drug that could be taken internally. Both ara-A and ara-C operate by interfering with the DNA of the virus, thereby interrupting its ability to replicate. Global annual sales of these drugs exceed one hundred million dollars. Of course, the dollar value of these drugs is an incomplete measure of their value in alleviating human suffering. But, in this particular case, the value of the drugs inspired by ara-A and ara-C is priceless. According to David Newman, ara-A and ara-C were the stimulus for the successful treatment of the late twentieth century's most dreaded medical scourge.

In June 1981, the Centers for Disease Control (CDC) in Atlanta reported on a rare type of pneumonia suffered by several gay men in Atlanta. Shortly thereafter, the term "AIDS" was coined to denote a disease characterized by a total collapse of the body's immune system. By 1987, the disease was found on every continent with the exception of Antarctica. By the early 1990s, the disease had infected millions of people and had killed cultural icons like Rudolf Nureyev, Rock Hudson, and Arthur Ashe.

AIDS has proven remarkably resilient in resisting Western medicine's most common preventative for viral diseases: vaccines.

In March 1987, however, the FDA approved a new drug for the treatment of AIDS: zidovudine, better known as AZT. The drug slowed the progress of the disease but did not stop it. In December 1995, the FDA approved the use of the protease inhibitor saquinavir (Invirase), which, when used with AZT and another chemical related to AZT, reduced the infected person's viral load to undetectable levels.

Newman has convincingly argued that AZT would never have been developed if it had not been for the odd chemicals extracted from Bergmann's Caribbean sponge. There can be no question that these led directly to ara-A and ara-C. Newman points out the chemical resemblance between these compounds and that of acyclovir, an antiviral drug in widespread use for the treatment of herpes. And acyclovir, he notes, was a precursor to the synthesis of AZT. In a recent technical paper co-authored with colleagues at the National Institutes of Health, Newman placed AZT in the category of what he calls "S*": "from a synthetic source, but originally modeled on a natural product parent." And Newman also notes that the protease inhibitor in the AIDS cocktail is also based on natural compounds!

Sponges from around the world are yielding a dazzling array of new compounds with medicinal potential. The little-known *Lissodendoryx* sponge, found only on a small section of reef off the coast of New Zealand, produces halichondrin B, a promising anticancer compound. Extracts of an Australian species show potential as a new treatment for falciparum malaria, one of the most lethal and drug-resistant strains of this dreaded disease. Another sponge yields compounds known as topsentins, anti-inflammatories that can be employed in the treatment of sunburns and even arthritis. Extracts of the bright red *Batzella* sponge from the Caribbean inhibit the replication of the HIV virus in the test tube.

Discodermolide, derived from yet another deep-water Caribbean sponge, offers exceptional promise. It first attracted scientists' attention because, in the test tube, the compound proved extremely effective as an immunosuppresant—it was one thousand times more potent than cyclosporin, and appeared to accomplish this through a different mechanism than the fungi-derived compound. Discodermolide exhibits potent anticancer activity and has proven at least as effective as the cancer drug taxol in treating breast and lung cancer and is eighty times as potent against leukemia cells. Further testing is now underway at the National Cancer Institute.

Not surprisingly, new cancer drugs are also being developed from marine creatures other than sponges. Diazonomide A, derived from a rare species of sea squirt discovered by Fenical in an underwater cave near the Filipino island of Siquijor, has proven effective at killing colon cancer cells in the test tube. Dolastatin 10, from the peculiar sea hare, a distant relative of the octopus, also offers anticancer potential and is being investigated in the lab. Bryozoans, nondescript creatures known as "moss animals," yield a compound being tested as a treatment of lymphoma, melanoma, and nephroma, three of the deadliest cancers. The drug, called bryostatin, functions by encouraging the body's immune system to attack the malignancy and by stimulating the activity of a protein that regulates the growth of cancer cells. Bryostatin is currently in phase 2 trials in both Europe and the States, meaning that it is already being tested on human subjects, with some degree of success. Of all the anticancer marine compounds under study, bryostatin is the most advanced and the most likely to make it to market in the short term.

Some marine creatures are medically important for reasons other than the chemicals they produce. Coral plays a surprising role in modern medicine. Physicians have long sought a substance that can substitute for human bone, but problems abound. The first hindrance: matching Mother Nature's engineering genius. Human bone is strong and supple, tough but porous. When metal substances are surgically implanted as bone replacement, the body's immune system often rejects the foreign substance. Doctors can take bone from one part of the body and move it to another to prevent rejection. This is exceedingly painful, however, and only small amounts of bone can be transplanted in this manner. And even this procedure can lead to infection. Twenty years ago, doctors began working with a near-perfect substitute for human bone: coral.

On a cumulative basis, coral reefs are probably the largest structures on earth built by nonhuman creatures: more than two hundred thousand tons of reefs are produced each year by tiny invertebrates called polyps, which manufacture the calcium carbonate structures in which they live. Once the original polyps have been cleaned out, the coral is almost protein-free, so it can be implanted in the human body without triggering an attack from the immune system. And the holes in the coral once inhabited by the tiny creatures serve as a tunnel system that can be traversed and filled both by human capillaries and by bone-building cells known as osteoblasts. The coral itself is slowly degraded by osteoblast cells, but the osteoblasts continue to deposit new bone to replace it.

The major drawbacks to using coral as a bone substitute is that the marine material shatters relatively easily. Coral is therefore not suitable for joint replacements, the most important type of bone replacement (more than half a million hips are replaced each year). As is so often the case with natural products, researchers have been studying how coral is formed to learn to produce a better synthetic bone substitute.

Meanwhile, scientists in Australia are developing new sunscreens from coral. Realizing that coral polyps receive enormous doses of ultraviolet radiation each day, they decided to investigate. The result: two patents on protective chemicals that may find their way into tanning lotions, sunscreens, and possibly even cosmetics.

Another denizen of the deep that plays a significant role in modern medicine is the peculiar horseshoe crab, which is more closely related to spiders than crustaceans. The hard, thick brown shell that covers most of the creature is horseshoe-shaped, hence its name. The shell terminates in a long spine. Underneath, the creature has six pairs of legs, giving it a bizarre and somewhat frightening appearance (despite its peaceful nature, the horseshoe crab was the model for the juvenile form of the murderous space creature in the film *Alien*). Nonetheless, the common species of horseshoe crab has proven to be one of the most medically useful animals ever studied.

Because these animals are relatively primitive in evolutionary terms compared to mammals, they have organ systems that are easier to study and comprehend. For example, the human eye is one of the most exceedingly complex organs in existence. Much of the understanding of how it functions in vision was actually realized by studies of the eyes of horseshoe crabs. By focusing on these arthropods, biophysicist Dr. Haldan Hartline conducted pioneering studies of how the eye converts visual stimulation into images, research that won him the Nobel Prize in 1967.

A major obstacle facing the developers of the first injectable medicines like penicillin was the presence of impurities called pyrogens, which caused high fever in the patients. Research at the Woods Hole Marine Biological Laboratory in Massachusetts found that the blood of the horseshoe crab readily coagulates in the presence of both bacterial toxins like pyrogens and several potentially lethal bacterial diseases like meningitis. This discovery led to the development and commercialization of the limulus amebocyte lysate test for pyrogens in pharmaceutical products and for gram-negative bacterial diseases like spinal meningitis and toxic shock syndrome.

Ironically, former senator William Proxmire, the self-appointed spending watchdog who gave one of his Golden Fleece Awards to the scientist who carried out seminal research on fireflies (as we saw in Chapter 4), made a similar blunder with respect to research on the horseshoe crab. William Sargent, who wrote a wonderful book about the horseshoe crab, suggested that Proxmire be presented with a "leaden *Limulus* for shortsightedness in the pursuit of government economy."

Perhaps no research project better exemplifies both the potential of new medicines from the sea—and the environmental crises that threaten them—than an ongoing effort by Dr. William Gerwick of Oregon State University. Intrigued by a blue-green algae name *Lyngba majuscula*, known to cause a severe skin rash upon contact, Gerwick initiated field work on this species near the Caribbean island of Curaçao. The scientist was surprised to find that one population of this algae lacked the chemicals known to cause the skin rash, but harbored two new immunosuppressive compounds, macrolin A and macrolin B. Then he found that this particular population also contained two new fish poisons and a novel snail poison. The latter he named barbamide, which he then tested in the lab where he found it a potent killer of snails that carry the dreaded disease schistosomiasis. As if this was not enough, Gerwick then isolated still another new compound from this same algae. Called curacin A, the compound exhibits potent activity against breast, colon, and kidney cancer, and it operates in a fashion similar to, but slightly different than, the periwinkle alkaloids. Because of this, according to natural product chemist Dr. Brad Carte at the pharmaceutical company Smith Kline Beecham, "[Curacin A] opens the door for the potential development of a new class of anti-cancer drugs."

The bad news, however, is that only the algae from the island's Spanish Lagoon produce these potential wonder drugs; other populations do not. Private developers are interested in building a gigantic housing development and golf course on the banks of the lagoon. According to Gerwick, who is collaborating with local environmentalists to prevent the project from moving forward, "If this development goes through, it will wipe out the algae—and who knows what else?"

Chapter Eight

PLANTS
OF THE APES

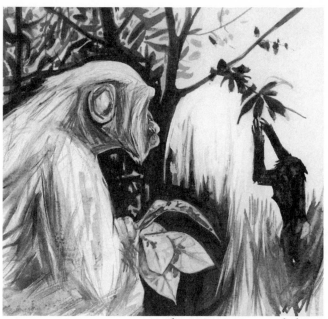

Chimpanzee (*Pan troglodytes*)

Do other species use plants to fight disease the way humans do? If so, the history of plant medicines could be older than the history of mankind.

—Dr. W. Acosta, 1996

In the summer of 1980, I had the opportunity to wander in the once great forests of eastern Brazil. The early European explorers were awestruck by the beauty and diversity of these woodlands, which stretched in an enormous unbroken arc from the easternmost tip of Brazil hundreds of miles south into what is now Paraguay and northern Argentina. However, what remains is a fragment of what once was: small isolated pockets of forest, home to a handful of plants and animals trying to hang on to an ever shrinking handhold: more than 96 percent of the original forest cover has been destroyed. And as I wandered through those distant patches of jungle, the sounds of trucks, bulldozers, radios, and human voices surrounded me on all sides, a constant reminder that our civilization was in the final throes of obliterating the little that was left.

The forest itself seemed almost empty; the large terrestrial creatures like the jaguar and the peccary that characterize the South American rain forest had been hunted out so thoroughly that I saw not even a pair of footprints. The haunting calls of the toucans and the piercing screeches of the macaws had long been stilled. Of course, these spectacular animals were not the only components that had been eliminated from these forests. In the course of preparing for my trip, I had combed the early accounts of the first Portuguese explorers who had ventured into these jungles almost five hundred years earlier; their reports were replete with tales of the warriors who once dominated this complex landscape. Though the jungle had been reduced by over 90 percent of its original range, tribes like the Botocudos and the Tupinikin had been completely exterminated.

What is the medical legacy of these Indians, and the once great forests in which they thrived? The Amazon jungle has provided us with ipecac and tubocurarine; tropical Africa has given us physostigmine and strophanthin; and the rain forests of Asia have yielded ajmaline and reserpine. Each of these medicines is derived from plants observed in use by local tribespeople. No major medical compound has ever been developed from an eastern Brazilian rain forest plant, and that is undoubtedly because the Botocudos and other tribes were obliterated before any ethnobotanical studies were ever conducted with them.

Without indigenous people to guide us, how best to determine which plants merit laboratory investigation? Of the sixteen parks and protected areas in Suriname, for example, twelve have no Indians living within the boundaries or nearby, a situation increasingly common in the tropics. If we are to find the new and useful compounds that do occur in the plants, how best to proceed?

American aviators preparing to fly over the jungles of Indochina during the Second World War were taught that the best way to survive if shot down was to "eat what the monkeys eat." While the overarching value of this advice was probably psychological (some monkeys have chambered stomachs capable of digesting leaves that would poison and possibly kill a human), this recommendation may ultimately prove more beneficial for medicinal purposes. For we are learning that, in many cases, instinct has programmed animals with an inherent knowledge of medicinal plants that our own species is only now beginning to appreciate and to study. A most extraordinary example comes from research on an endangered species of primate in the Atlantic forest of eastern Brazil.

In the early 1980s, Karen Strier, a Harvard graduate student in biological anthropology, traveled to the eastern Brazilian state of Minas Gerais to conduct research on monkeys in their natural habitat. She chose as her study site the farm of Feliciano Miguel Abdala, a rancher who had established a four-square-mile private forest reserve on his land, home to a thriving population of muriquis (also known as woolly spider monkeys), the largest and most apelike of the New World monkeys. Strier's studies soon led her to some surprising conclusions. The diet of muriquis proved much higher in tannins than those of other monkeys. Because tannins comprise about 50 percent of the antidysentery drug Enterovioform, the Harvard scientist wondered if the primates were modifying their diets to kill parasites or control the diarrhea that often accompanies parasite infestation. Subsequent investigation revealed that the muriquis in this forest were completely free of parasites—highly unusual for a rain forest primate. And several of these plants are identical to (or closely related to) species taken by Amazonian Indians to control parasites.

Prior to the onset of the breeding season, Strier noted that the muriqui's diet consisted primarily of the leaves of two tree species rich in antimicrobial compounds. During that same time of year, the monkeys visit the monkey's ear tree (so named because of the shape of the fruits) to feed. As a general rule, when monkeys find trees laden with edible fruit, they gorge themselves until little remains. Yet Strier wrote that the muriquis consumed a small portion of the fruits before departing "as if they only need a taste to be satisfied." Once back at Harvard, she learned that these fruits are rich in stimasterol, a chemical employed in the manufacture of progesterone, which is itself used in birth control pills. Plant hormones can affect animal fertility. Did the monkeys of this forest discover the birth control pills tens of thousands of years before their human cousins did?

Primatologist Dr. Ken Glander of Duke University has spent decades studying the howler monkeys of Central America and has reached conclusions that parallel those of Karen Strier. Glander hypothesizes that the howler monkeys *eat a selection of plants that allows them to select the sex of their offspring!* He notes that female howlers consume certain plants before and after copulation that they do not eat at any other time. Over two decades of study,

Glander found that some howlers bore only male offspring, while others produced only females, an outcome unlikely due to chance. "Female" sperm (those that carry an X chromosome) do better than "male" sperm (which carry a Y chromosome) in an acidic environment—and vice versa. Could female howlers be controlling the chemistry of their reproductive tract and, if so, why? Glander suggests that plant-derived estrogen-like chemicals may be responsible. He notes that males in a monkey troop often pass more of their genes to the next generation than females are able to do. This would explain why it is often advantageous for a female to produce more males or, if there already exists a surfeit of males, why female offspring are preferable.

The study of how animals use plants for medicinal purposes has recently been termed "zoopharmacognosy"—but our observation of this phenomenon is, without question, an ancient practice. Who has not watched a dog swallow grass to induce vomiting when the animal has eaten something unhealthy it wishes to regurgitate? In a thought-provoking research paper, the brilliant ecologist Dr. Dan Janzen of the University of Pennsylvania wrote, "I would like to ask if plant-eating vertebrates may do it on occasion as a way of writing their own prescriptions."

Sometimes animals teach us by their wisdom, other times by their foolishness. Fatal culinary errors made by North American cows in the early part of the twentieth century led to the development of several blockbuster drugs. One Saturday afternoon in February 1933 in the middle of a howling blizzard, a Wisconsin farmer appeared in the office of chemist Dr. Karl Link carrying a bucket of blood. The man had driven almost two hundred miles from his farm near Deer Park to seek help from the state veterinarian headquartered at the University of Wisconsin in Madison. It was the weekend, however, and the vet's office was closed, so the desperate farmer wandered into the first building he found where the door was not locked: the biochemistry building.

The blood in the bucket he carried would not clot. Several of his cows had recently hemorrhaged to death, and now his bull was oozing blood from the nose. He had been feeding his herd with the only hay he had: spoiled sweet clover.

This hemorrhagic disease had first been reported in the 1920s from both North Dakota and Alberta, Canada. While specialists determined that feeding the animals spoiled sweet clover was the cause of this malady, they were not able to cure it, nor were they able to isolate the compound in the clover that caused the problem. Their recommendation: destroy the spoiled forage and transfuse healthy blood into the hemorrhaging cattle, the same advice offered by Link. Unfortunately, however, the farmer lacked an alternative fodder to feed his herd, and he was unable to perform blood transfusions in rural Wisconsin during the Depression.

Troubled by his inability to assist, Link mentioned the problem to German postdoctoral student Eugene W. Schoeffel. Schoeffel, an emotional and idealistic man fond of quoting Goethe and Shakespeare, undertook the spoiled clover conundrum as a personal crusade. He and his colleagues analyzed the clover for seven years before identifying and isolating the cause of its lethality: a chemical they named dicumarol. They correctly hypothesized that if too much caused a hemorrhage, a minuscule amount might prove to be a useful anticoagulant. Today, dicumarol (and its synthetic analogues) are commonly employed as anticoagulants, particularly for the prevention and treatment of pulmonary embolism and venous thrombosis.

The clover analysis serves as yet another example in which a single species yields a multitude of products. Noticing that one of the synthetic analogues seemed to induce particularly severe bleeding in rodents, Link proposed testing it as a rat poison, thinking it might lack the obvious dangers of more toxic rodenticides like strychnine. Research on this compound was bankrolled by the Wisconsin Alumni Research Foundation; when proved effective, it was named warfarin. (Despite the bellicose connotations, the name came from the acronym of the alumni group!)

In early 1951, an army inductee tried to commit suicide by eating warfarin. He failed to kill himself but did manage to induce a classic case of hemorrhagic sweet clover syndrome. The unhappy soldier was successfully treated with transfusions of normal blood and coagulants. This bizarre incident led to studies and eventual approval of warfarin (renamed coumadin) as an anticoagulant for human patients. How many cardiac patients realize that their physicians are prescribing rat poison for their ills?

Yet another aspect of animal behavior has led us to other therapeutic leads. A surprisingly wide variety of creatures ingest and store toxic natural compounds in their own bodies. They do this not for medicinal purposes, but to employ the poisons for their own purposes, either to equip themselves with the ability to deliver a poisonous bite, or to deter predators from eating them. This is the case with the poisonous pufferfish.

A deadly nerve poison, tetrodotoxin, occurs in dozens of pufferfish species. These fish concentrate the poison in their internal organs. Though the logical correlation is that humans would go to great lengths to avoid these toxic denizens of the deep, pufferfish are considered a delicacy in Japan. Chefs must undergo special training and then be licensed by the federal government before being permitted to prepare this sought-after delicacy. Despite the rigorous preparation, accidents do happen: every few years, someone is poisoned. The result: general numbness, loss of muscle control, and, unless treated, death. Intrigued by the numbness typical of tetrodotoxin envenomation, Japanese physicians have used it as a treatment for pain caused by migraines or menstrual cramps.

Scientists were surprised to find that the deadly bite of the blue-ringed octopus contained tetrodotoxin. Was it possible that the pufferfish and the octopus were creating the same poison? They found that neither the fish nor the octopus was capable of producing the poison—a microbe known as *Vibrio* manufactured it. The fish and the mollusk were ingesting the microbe and then storing the poison in their internal organs to deter predators. In a way, the puffer and the octopus had done our research for us—of the millions of microbes in the sea, they had found one of the deadliest (with potent medical applications) and brought it to our attention, albeit in a most fatal fashion.

Not only are animals helping find new chemicals, they are helping us produce them in the lab. Dr. Shirley Pomponi, the director of biomedical marine research at Harbor Branch Oceanographic Institution in Fort Pierce, Florida, is a specialist on marine invertebrates investigating ecteinascidin (ECT), an antimelanoma compound mentioned in Chapter 7. "Unfortunately," said Pomponi, "it could take nearly a ton of sea squirts to produce a mere gram of ecteinascidin." Pomponi and her Harbor Branch colleagues found a flatworm that not only feeds on the sea squirt, but also filters and stores the ecteinascidin, presumably using the compound like the pufferfish uses tetrodotoxin—to make itself unpalatable to predators. The scientists have succeeded in developing a method of "milking" ECT from the flatworm that is much more cost effective than extracting it from the sea squirt.

This method of filching a poison from another species and using it for protection has helped us understand how dart poison frogs become so toxic. As we saw in Chapter 1, tropical American dart frogs contain myriad fascinating chemical compounds. Until recently, however, we were unable to determine how the frogs made the poison. When raised in captivity, these amphibians often failed to produce the same toxins. Specimens captured in the wild and placed in captivity may keep their alkaloids. But their progeny have fewer or none of these alkaloids.

Hawaii produced an even stranger phenomenon. Poison dart frogs were released in the Manoa Valley on the island of Oahu in 1932. When the descendants of these amphibian immigrants were tested in the lab fifty years after the original introduction, scientists found two of the same types of alkaloids that occur in the original species (which is native to Panama). Another type of alkaloid found in the Panamanian species was absent. And scientists found a new alkaloid in the Hawaiian frog that does not occur in the Panamanian version! What is going on here?

Poison dart frog authority Dr. John Daly hypothesized that: (1) the amphibians make the alkaloids themselves; (2) they made the alkaloids from something that they consumed; or (3) they collected and stored the compounds from a component of their diet, much as the pufferfish does with tetrodotoxin. The answer to Daly's hypothesis seems to be a combination of all three. Some of the compounds (or their precursors) are found in insects eaten by the frog: alkaloids are taken in and stored from beetles, ants, and millipedes. But it was not just a question of ingesting and sequestering any and all alkaloids: when ants containing two different alkaloids were fed to the frogs, the little amphibians stored only one alkaloid in their skin and apparently excreted the other. And, in some instances, the frogs were observed seeking out and consuming particular species of insects that harbored compounds that the frogs typically stored in their own skin. Thus the painkiller ABT-594, currently being developed by Abbott Labs, supposedly from a frog poison, may actually be based on an insect poison that was presented to us by the frog!

In terms of intentionally using plants for medicinal purposes, the great apes of Africa are the most sophisticated members of the animal kingdom. Harvard primatologist Dr. Richard Wrangham observed chimpanzees in Uganda's Kibale Forest consuming a tropical daisy called *Aspilia* in the early 1980s. While chimps devour most of the plants in their largely vegetarian diet, Wrangham made note of the unusual behavior surrounding consumption of this species: the leaves were carefully chosen and then swallowed. Furthermore, the primates' faces appeared to indicate severe distaste, like a child taking castor oil. Because chimps, like people, are prone to parasitic infections, Wrangham hypothesized that the monkeys were consuming these leaves for medicinal (rather than nutritional) purposes.

Wrangham brought *Aspilia* to the lab for analysis and received startling results: the plant contained a novel compound (they named it thiarubrine) that proved to have potent antibiotic, fungicidal, and vermicidal properties. Curiously, they also learned that this plant and related species are widely employed by African peoples for a panoply of medicinal uses: from treating cuts to cystitis to gonorrhea. This in turn raised another issue: was it the use of this plant by the chimps that led people to experiment with it in the first place?

Ethnobotanists—scientists who study peoples' use of local plants—have long wondered how a culture learns which species harbor medicinal qualities. While the process of trial and error clearly plays a significant role in this process, might not the plants employed by animals offer a natural starting place for experimentation?

The thiarubrine story had a bizarre footnote: when scientists retested *Aspilia* in the lab, they only found thiarubrine in the roots of the plant, which the chimps do not eat. African, European, Japanese, and American research teams have repeatedly confirmed that the primates consume only the leaves. Why, then, are parasite-ridden chimps eating the leaves? Primatologist Dr. Michael Huffman, an American scientist who lives in Japan and works in Tanzania, found the answer in an ingenious bit of field research. Huffman and his colleagues found that the chimps' droppings often contained both *Aspilia* leaves and intestinal worms that had been impaled on stiff tiny hairs (known as trichomes) on the leaf surface. Though the chimps were taking the leaves as "medicine," it was not a chemical that killed the parasite, but a physical remedy that simply scraped out and lanced the offending organism. Huffman christened this process the "Velcro effect." Because of this research, however, scientists had indeed discovered a new antibiotic.

Huffman, who was inspired to choose a career in primatology by his childhood fascination with H. A. Rey's *Curious George*, eventually collected concrete evidence that the chimps were employing other plants as chemical medicines rather than just botanical Velcro. Huffman has focused much of his field research in the Mahale region of Tanzania along the eastern shore of Lake Tanganyika, close to where the explorer Stanley found David Livingstone more than a century ago (and about one hundred miles north of Jane Goodall's famous site at Gombe Stream). There, Huffman's guide and mentor is Mohamedi Seifu Kalunde, a soft-spoken elder of the local WaTongwe tribe. Kalunde is both a skilled naturalist and a renowned herbalist. Kalunde and Huffman were tracking a sick female chimp in November 1987 when the chimp stopped in front of a *Vernonia* bush of the daisy family, tore off a branch, and began peeling the bark. Ten years later, Huffman still vividly recalls the events that transpired: "Mohamedi said, 'That is very strange. I don't know why she is eating that because it is very bitter.' I asked 'Do they eat it a lot?' and he said 'No.' Then I asked him if his people made use of it and he said, 'Yes. We take it for stomach problems.' "

Vernonia represents one of the most important and widely used medicinal plants of the African continent. In Ethiopia, it is valued as a treatment for malaria; people in South Africa value it for amoebic dysentery. Tribespeople in Zaire use it for diarrhea, and the Angolans utilize it for upset stomach. In Kitongwe, the language of Huffman's guide and mentor, Kalunde, the name for *Vernonia* is *njonso*, which means both "bitterleaf" and "the real medicine."

As they watched the sick chimp, she finished peeling the bark and began chewing on the stem. She did not swallow it, however, but spit out the chewed remains, only ingesting the bitter sap. Huffman doubts the sap is an "acquired taste" consumed for gustatory purposes—the flavor is exceptionally foul. (The great Jane Goodall performed an intriguing experiment, which probably has some bearing on Huffman's observation: when she gave sick chimps bananas laced with the antibiotic tetracycline, they readily devoured them. However, when she offered the same drug-laden fruits to healthy chimps, they refused them.) Huffman and Kalunde continued to follow the sick chimp, which made a rapid recovery. Prior to consuming the plant sap, the chimp was suffering from constipation, malaise, and lack of appetite. A day later, she had made a spectacular recovery: the researchers had trouble keeping her in sight as she began climbing ridges at a rapid clip.

Of course, a single observation of a single sick chimp cannot be considered convincing proof in and of itself. Yet in December 1991, the research team made similar observations that added credence to their theory. Huffman and Kalunde observed another sick chimp eating *Vernonia* and managed to test their hypothesis. As they tracked the chimp, they collected samples of her droppings for laboratory analysis. At the time of the first collection, the stools contained 130 nematode eggs per gram. Less than twenty-four hours later, the egg level was reduced to 15 per gram and the chimp had resumed hunting, an energy-intensive exercise that she appeared unable to perform the day before. When the researchers calculated exactly how much of the plant the animal had ingested, they found that her dosage was almost identical to that taken by ailing tribespeople. The period of recovery—twenty to twenty-four hours— was identical for both people and chimps. And though the plant was common and available year round, chimps tended to consume it only during the rainy season, when parasite infections are most prevalent.

Working with Japanese colleagues, Huffman had the plant chemically analyzed. Lab work revealed two types of chemical compounds that accounted for the plant's medicinal use. The plants are rich in sesquiterpene lactones, chemicals found in many botanical species and known to have antihelminthic (antiworm), antiamoebic, and antibiotic properties. New sesquiterpene lactones found in these plants demonstrated significant activity against leishmaniasis (a common and disfiguring tropical disease) as well as drug-resistant falciparum malaria.

Appropriately, the first commercial use of these *Vernonia* extracts may be for animals rather than people. Huffman has been collaborating with colleagues in both Denmark and Tanzania to determine the efficacy of *Vernonia* extracts in killing a nematode known by the scientific name *Osteophagostum stephanostomum* (another instance in which the name is longer than the creature itself!). These nematodes (and their close relatives) cause significant loss of livestock, particularly in the tropical world. Current treatments, while effective, are often expensive by Third World standards, and inaccessible. The quality of livestock husbandry in the tropics could be vastly improved by providing farmers with a plant they can grow and use to kill parasites safely and effectively.

Even if developed successfully, *Vernonia* would not represent the first example of a useful tropical plant finding its way into the medicine cabinet of the veterinarian rather than the physician. The fruit of the betel palm is the stimulant of choice in many parts of Asia, where local peoples chew it wrapped in a leaf of a local pepper vine. Alkaloids in the fruit provide a chemical stimulus, and some claim that betel is as addictive as tobacco. Several decades ago, chemists isolated an alkaloid from the palm, which they called "arecoline" because the scientific name for the palm genus is *Areca*. Although initially used by physicians as a human vermifuge (an antiparasitic agent), arecoline was eventually judged too toxic for our own species and is currently employed as a treatment for parasites in animals.

Animals often prove "tougher" than humans do; they don't suffer the side effects some drugs cause in people. Few animals live as long as our species, so they won't incur the deleterious effects that may result from taking a drug for many decades.

Hence, many of the drugs (both natural and synthetic) currently in development will be used for animals instead of people (or for both). The magnitude of the veterinary market is enormous, encompassing everything from domestic dogs and cats to zoo animals to cattle, pigs, sheep, and horses that serve as the bases for agricultural operations all over the world. The annual retail value of veterinary drugs for the U.S. market is one billion dollars.

But some plants harbor compounds potentially useful both for human and veterinary medicine. Fig trees dominate some tropical forests, where their fruits serve as major dietary components for both birds and primates. Chimps use the trees for medicinal purposes as well as food. In the western Amazon, the sap of one species is so highly valued as a cure for parasitic infections that it is bottled and sold commercially. The leaves of an African species are eaten by chimps in Tanzania probably because they contain enzymes that kill nematodes, chimpanzees' most common intestinal parasites. The young leaves—which the chimps eat—contain 600 percent more of the antiparasitic agent than do the older fig leaves.

Fig sap is also consumed medicinally by another large mammal: the elephant. Presumably these pachyderms value it for its antiparasitic nature, much as local peoples use the plant. But fig trees aren't the only medicinal plant consumed by the elephants. In the early 1940s, scientists observed Asian elephants devouring the fruits of the legume *Entada scheffleri* before embarking on lengthy treks, leading researchers to hypothesize that the plant may serve as either a stimulant or a painkiller (or could it merely be pachyderm carbo-loading?). World Wildlife Fund ecologist Dr. Holly Dublin spent much of 1975 tracking and observing a pregnant elephant in Tsavo Park in southern Kenya. The elephant had a standard routine of covering about three miles a day in search of edible plants. One day, the mother-to-be walked almost twenty miles and devoured an entire tree of the borage family. Dublin never observed this creature eat this species before or after this particular incident. Four days later, the elephant gave birth.

While this may not initially seem to be cause and effect, Dublin soon stumbled across an interesting connection: pregnant women in Kenya prepare and consume a tea of the bark and leaves of this species to induce either labor or abortion! When Michael Huffman related this story to Kalunde, the Kenyan replied that his grandfather had taught him that WaTongwe women had used this plant for the same purpose in the past. Huffman noted that the WaTongwe live in southwestern Tanzania, more than one hundred miles south of Tsavo, implying that the custom was probably the case in more than one elephant individual or population.

According to Huffman, Mohamedi learned most of what he knows about medicinal plants from his late grandfather, who gleaned insight into the potential utility of the flora by observing the behavior of the local fauna. Kalunde related the tale of a sick African crested porcupine that dug up and consumed the roots of a local plant known as *mulengelele*. The little creature soon recovered from bouts of diarrhea and lethargy, often the symptoms of a parasite infestation. Kalunde claimed that this led the WaTongwe to begin employing *mulengelele* to treat parasite infestations among themselves. Huffman cautions that this story may be merely an "interesting teaching device" to pass important information down from one generation to another, and adds that medicinal plant use has never before been reported in porcupines. Can we afford to dismiss this as an allegorical tale for transmitting information to children and grandchildren, or should *mulengelele* be investigated in the lab?

This episode parallels an experience I had in the northeast Amazon with an extraordinary tribal group known as the Maroons. When slaves were brought to the Amazon in the seventeenth and eighteenth centuries, many managed to escape from captivity into the rain forest. There they coalesced into tribal societies very much patterned on the African cultures from which they had been forcibly removed. They were warriors perhaps by nature but certainly by necessity, as they represented a severe threat to the plantation economy of the local colonies. (As long as there was a "home" in the forest for runaway slaves, servants on the plantation were that much more likely to take up arms and/or escape.) In Brazil, the Maroons managed to organize themselves into the city-state known as Palmares, which was eventually razed to the ground by white plantation owners and their henchmen. In Suriname, however, the Maroons were never conquered, and there these unique African-American cultures continue to thrive.

From an ethnobotanical perspective, the Maroons are exceedingly interesting in that they have an origin in and a relationship with the forest different from that of the local Indians. For example, they employ some plants for medicinal purposes that the Amerindians do not use. Because the Indians have lived in the forest for thousands of years and the Maroons have only been there several hundred years, it is tempting to assume that the latter know much less about the forest because they are relatively recent arrivals. I came to find out that this is not always the case.

I was visiting the capital of Paramaribo, sitting on the terrace of a bar overlooking the muddy brown Suriname River that flows gently past the city. With me was Chris Healy, an American raised in Suriname who is an expert on Maroon art and culture. We were speaking about people, plants, and animals of the forest when he told me an exceedingly peculiar tale about the tapir, the largest mammal of the Amazon forest. According to Chris, the Maroons claim that tapirs eat the stems of the *nekoe* plant, defecate into forest streams, and eat the fish that rise to the surface, stunned by compounds in the plants. In fact, *nekoe* (known elsewhere in Latin America as *barbasco*) does contain chemicals known as rotenoids that interfere with fishes' ability to intake oxygen, causing them to float to the surface if *nekoe* has been added to the water in which they swim. Local peoples (both Indians and Maroons) take advantage of this phenomenon by throwing crushed *nekoe* stems into the river and catching the fish that rise to the surface. This plant serves as the source of rotenone, which is used as a biodegradable pesticide by organic gardeners and was valued by American soldiers during the Second World War to kill mites that had infested their clothing.

Thinking that the Indians know more about the forest and its creatures than the Maroons do, I queried several Amerindian colleagues about tapirs and *nekoe*, but they steadfastly denied any connection between the two. However, every Maroon that I asked told me that tapirs eat *nekoe*, defecate the remains in forest streams, and so on. Does this mean that the Maroons learned of the fish-stunning capabilities of *nekoe* from watching tapirs? Or is this merely something on the order of a fanciful tale concocted to teach youngsters about the value of the vine, much as Huffman suggests may have been the case with the *mulengelele* and the African crested porcupine?

One of the reasons to suspect that the Maroons may well have learned from the tapirs is that so much more evidence of animal use of medicinal plants has come to light since scientists began looking for it over the course of the previous decade. Chimps are the best-documented group in terms of plant use for medicinal purposes. (It may be argued that their utilization of healing plants is somehow not particularly representative of the animal kingdom as a whole because these primates are so closely related to us: our DNA is more than 95 percent identical to that of chimps; chimps are more closely related to us than they are to the other great apes [gorillas and orangutans], and blood transfusions between people and chimps are said to be theoretically possible.) The great apes are known to employ over thirty species of plants for medicinal purposes. This may well represent what scientists term an "artifact of collection," meaning that the most attractive and conspicuous animals receive the most attention, hence we conclude that these species use more medicinal plants than other creatures.

In fact, the more we look, the more we find. Even the literature contains a long and extensive list of animals (mostly mammals, probably for reasons noted above) consuming botanicals for purposes that are presumably therapeutic. Pigs are notoriously prone to parasitic worm infestations, and wild boars in both India and Mexico often consume plants with known antihelminthic properties: pigweed in India and pomegranate roots in Mexico. Yet, there's an unusual twist to this pig story. In India, local people extract and utilize a worm-killing medicine from the pigweed roots. But though pomegranate root bark is known to contain an alkaloid that kills tapeworms, neither the pig nor the pomegranate is native to Mexico: the Spanish conquistadors brought both to the New World. The pigs nonetheless selectively seek out and consume the roots of this tree as their ancestors once did in the Old World.

In the course of his research, Dan Janzen of the University of Pennsylvania unearthed a paper published in 1939 that noted that the Asian two-horned rhino was observed eating so much of the tannin-rich bark of the red mangrove that its urine was stained bright orange. Tannins are a major component of some over-the-counter antidiarrheal preparations such as Enterovioform. Janzen has noted that the concentration of tannins in the bladder of the rhino necessary to change the color of its urine was undoubtedly sufficient to have an impact on parasites in the creature's bladder or urinary tract.

These animal-plant interactions have also been observed outside the tropics. Dr. Shawn Sigstedt, a laconic, Harvard-trained ethnobotanist, has focused his studies on the plants, animals, and peoples of the American West. Sigstedt's favorite plants are a small genus of herbs known as *Ligusticum*, but he is not the only one captivated by this somewhat nondescript little plant. When bears encounter the plant, they exhibit peculiar behavior: *Ligusticum* functions as an ursine catnip. Sigstedt once observed *Ligusticum* roots thrown into a brown-bear zoo enclosure, and a brawl ensued. The victor carried the roots to a corner of the cage, chewed them up, spit them out, and rubbed them all over his face and body. Both grizzlies and polar bears have proven similarly enamored of this little plant.

The Navajos of northern Arizona taught Sigstedt that the name for *Ligusticum* in their language translated into English means "bear medicine." These Indians value this plant as a treatment for many different ailments, treatments whose effectiveness is borne out by chemical analysis that documented the presence of compounds that are anticoagulant and antibacterial, as well as other chemicals that may combat both fungi and insect vermin. To these Indians, the bear is a sacred creature; in their creation tales, these animals are considered experts in the use of medicines.

Sigstedt is a bit surprised that his findings were considered so astonishing when he began reporting them in the late 1980s. "After all," he said, "deer and elk have long been known to chew aspen bark that contains compounds similar to aspirin. Why should bears be any less adept at using plants than these creatures?" He also feels that people's amazement upon discovering that bears were using these plants may have more to do with our perception and categorization than with that of the animals. "We tend to make a clear distinction between what is a food and what is a medicine, but this may not be the case with animals. Why should something that is good for you be only nutritious rather than medicinal? We tend to place a somewhat artificial barrier between food and medicine where the actual situation is probably better described as a complex mosaic."

This epicurean animal behavior noted by Sigstedt has also been observed in tropical America. Coatimundis, long-nosed relatives of the raccoon, have been observed rubbing the resin of a tropical relative of myrrh into their fur, presumably to kill or repel lice, mosquitoes, ticks, or other noxious vermin. The capuchin monkeys of tropical America (which used to be known as "organ grinder monkeys" because they were the species of choice for Italian-American organ grinders at the turn of the century) have similar practices but are known to utilize a wider variety of plant species. Capuchins have been observed rubbing eight different plants into their fur. Of these, four (*Hymenaea*, *Piper*, *Protrium*, and *Virola*) rank among the most common medicinal plants used by Amazonian Indians, and at least two of these are used by the Native Americans to treat skin problems.

Capuchins in Costa Rica massage a mixture of *Hymenaea* resin and rain water into their fur. The Suriname Maroons collect this same dried resin and make it into a tea to treat diarrhea, or burn it to keep away flying insects. Laboratory analysis has revealed that this resin harbors compounds that repel insects. American anthropologist Dr. Mary Baker observed these monkeys rubbing four other plant species into their fur. Peasants in the region use three related species to repel insects or treat skin problems.

Perhaps the most intriguing find of late is that birds appear to be making use of plants as both medicines and pesticides. Investigators were puzzled as to why penguins had almost no parasites or other harmful microorganisms in their digestive tract. Further field study revealed that the penguins were consuming blue-green algae on a regular basis and, as we saw in the previous chapter, these marine organisms are often loaded with potent chemical compounds (hence their use in experimental cancer therapy).

Researchers working in the Monte Verde Cloud Forest Reserve in western Costa Rica have recently reported an even more striking use of medicinal plants. This is one of the first protected areas established in Central America. More than twenty years ago, when this reserve was first declared, forest covered most of Costa Rica like a warm green blanket. Thanks to "development," most has been cleared; what remains exists primarily in national parks and other protected sites (yet the major source of foreign exchange in Costa Rica is ecotourism!).

Monte Verde, surrounded by a sea of deforested land, has become a mecca for both tourists and researchers looking for a study site that won't be converted into a smoking ruin. Though exceptionally rich in biodiversity, the Monte Verde region is devoid of indigenous tribespeople who might be able to teach us the medicinal value of the local flora. Like Karen Strier in eastern Brazil, two American researchers learned the therapeutic value of one Monte Verde plant from an animal rather than from an indigenous colleague.

Dr. K. Greg Murray and Dr. Kathy Winnett-Murray, a husband-and-wife team, have been studying the relationship between a small thrush known as the black-faced solitaire and a tiny red cousin of the tomato known as *Witheringia*, which tastes like a tomato but is much sweeter. Unlike most people, the Murrays are well aware that fruit represents something of a "contract" between frugivores (animals that eat fruit) and the plants themselves. Plants offer a tasty and nutritious food (the fruit) that the animals seek out and consume. In return, animals are "expected" to defecate the seeds (which are usually protected by indigestible seed coats) away from the plant that produced the fruit, thereby allowing the immobile plant to distribute its seeds away from the parent to a site where it will not compete for light and water. As is so often the case with negotiations, sometimes one of the parties manages to get the upper hand. The Murrays found that this is clearly the case with *Witheringia*, which is manipulating the solitaires to do its bidding far beyond what we would expect a plant to be capable of doing to a "sentient" being.

The Murrays reached their conclusions based on an exceedingly clever and elegant experiment. They began by creating two types of false fruits by using a red jelly that contained the *Witheringia* seeds. One batch was soaked in an extract of the real berries and was therefore impregnated with the chemicals found in the fruit. The other "fruits" consisted only of the jelly and the seeds. The scientists then presented the "fruits" to the hungry solitaires. Birds that ate the berries without the fruit extract excreted the seeds about twenty-five minutes after they ate. However, the solitaires that ate the berries soaked in the fruit extract defecated the seeds in only fifteen minutes, approximately the same amount of time it took them to excrete the seeds after eating the real fruits. The Murrays concluded that the fruit (and the fruit extract) contains a laxative that causes the birds to excrete the seeds one-third faster. While it may appear that the extra ten minutes the seeds spend in the bird's digestive system might not make any real difference, such is not the case. The Murrays found that 75 percent of the seeds that had spent only fifteen minutes in the birds were viable, whereas only 20 percent of seeds that spent ten minutes more inside the bird were able to germinate. Chemist Dr. William Acosta has suggested that this type of experiment (and these compounds in particular) could conceivably lead to the development of a new natural laxative for humans.

And birds use plants for other purposes, which could also lead us to new and useful compounds. Hawks have long been known to place sprigs of green leaves in their nests. Recently, birders have begun to notice that hawks select only the live branches of certain tree species and replace the dead or dying leaves with fresh material every few days. The red-tailed hawk uses the leaves of the cottonwood and quaking aspen, while the bald eagle chooses sedge and the needles of the white pine. In a classic study of this phenomenon, Dr. Bradley McDonald and his colleagues found that seven species of raptors (hawks and their relatives) were using over twelve species of plants. Though other scientists have advanced hypotheses to explain this behavior, from camouflaging the nest to advertising nest occupancy, McDonald's group tested these plants in the lab and found that all effectively repel insects (in this case, house flies, although they suggest that these leaves are also noxious to other vermin like mites as well as bacteria). Because these birds are carnivores, the adults regularly carry dead or dying creatures to the nest to feed their offspring. The blood and decomposing flesh of these prey items attract a steady stream of insects and bacteria that have the capacity to weaken and kill the young birds. By using the green plants that they do, the adult raptors protect their offspring in what is probably the first-known ornithological case of preventative medicine.

Compared to the trees of the temperate forest, the chemical

composition of rain forest tree leaves is relatively unstudied. In McDonald's study, he noted that antibacterial compounds had already been isolated from the leaves of one of these plant species before he began his study. Similar investigations of whether tropical birds employ local leaves for repellent and/or antibacterial purposes are now under way. But Neil Rettig, the foremost authority on the world's largest eagle, the Amazonian harpy, has already observed these magnificent creatures applying live branches of the giant *Mora* tree in their nests in a similar fashion. And what might be an insect repellent for the birds may one day prove to be a safe and effective insect repellent or antibiotic for us.

If we can find new painkillers from frogs, new stimulants from porcupines, new antiparasitics from penguins, new laxatives from thrushes, new antibiotics from chimps, and new contraceptives from woolly spider monkeys, what else might be out there, in the rain forest, on the prairie, or inside the coral reef, being used by local species and awaiting our discovery of its benefit to our own species? What might have already been lost? When the Portuguese first arrived on the eastern shores of Brazil almost five hundred years ago, the population of muriqui monkeys probably numbered in the hundreds of thousands. Now their population has been reduced to a few hundred individuals, and more than 90 percent of their once magnificent forests has been destroyed. Who knows what we lost, either in terms of the actual chemicals, the species that produced them, or the primate knowledge of how to use them?

Chapter Nine

SHAMANS

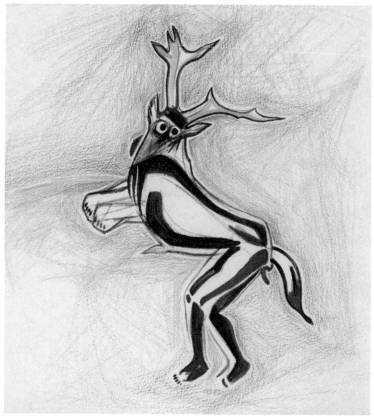

The Dancing Sorcerer of Trois Frères

Contrary to popular belief, the medicine man, or shaman (usually an accomplished botanist), represents the most ancient profession in the evolution of human culture.

—Dr. Richard Evans Schultes, 1963

He didn't look like a medicine man to me when I first met him.

Having been raised on a steady diet of Tarzan films, I first entered the rain forest expecting to find the medicine man (or "witch doctor") outfitted in full forest regalia: grass skirts, carnivore tooth necklaces, feather headdress. And indeed I did eventually work with shamans wearing even more fantastic costumes (or almost nothing, in some instances) when I entered the jungles of the northeast Amazon in the late 1970s. But as ever-encroaching Western civilization began making its appearance throughout the most remote corners of Amazonia, the young indigenous people lost interest in the old ways. Living in a world where the cultural global icons were people like Bruce Lee, Madonna, and Michael Jordan, the young Indians showed little or no interest in their own traditional cultures. The world of the shamans, with their belief in magic spirit worlds and astral travel, seemed less useful and effective than antibiotics. And if the missionaries or government-sponsored nurses insisted that shamanism was a sham, why pay any attention to a great-grandfather who said otherwise? So I would enter villages to find ancient wizards and plant masters wearing traditional breechcloths and jaguar-tooth necklaces but their descendants dressed in National Basketball Association T-shirts and high-top tennis shoes. In fifteen years of field experience, I had met few shamans who were not at least twice as old (and, more often, thrice as old) as I was.

But this fellow was different.

It was the first day of August, 1995, and I was seated in a cotton hammock under a thatched roof in the western Amazon of Colombia. To get there, I had to fly south from the Andean city of Bogotá to the burgeoning frontier town of Florencia, the capital city of the state of Caquetá; then an all-day bus ride past the military checkpoints and through the depressingly deforested landscape. In the 1960s, the national government, with the best of intentions, had encouraged landless peasants to settle on the "fertile" soils of the "uninhabited" Amazon region. The peasants' inability to manage the (admittedly challenging) tropical landscape resulted in forest destruction of staggering proportions. When my mentor Richard Schultes carried out ethnobotanical research here in the 1940s and 1950s, he marveled at "the seemingly limitless forest that stretched unbroken to the far horizon." Schultes returned to the area only a decade later, and writer William Burroughs was there to record the scientist's reaction: "My God, what have they done to the forest. . . . It's all gone!"

I had traveled to the area at the invitation of a Colombian colleague to participate in an ayahuasca ritual, the vision-vine ceremony conducted by Amazonian shamans for purposes of curing and divination. In South and North America, ayahuasca had attained an enormous and devoted following among certain New Age groups, though none of the practitioners whom I met were Native American shamans. The invitation to the Colombian Amazon seemed to represent the opportunity to participate in a truly traditional ceremony.

On that torrid afternoon, sweat poured off me and a few mosquitoes buzzed hungrily around my ears as I conversed with a fellow who stood leaning against the wooden post from which one end of my hammock was strung. He stood about five-foot-two, the typical height of a forest Indian, though the local campesinos (peasants) were not much taller. He had jet black hair and spoke excellent Spanish, again making it difficult for me to ascertain whether he was a Native American or not (knowing that such a question can be considered extremely rude by both cultures, I would not ask him outright). He took a last, long draught of his warm beer, and asked me if I'd ever been to the jungle before. I replied that I had worked in several South American countries searching for healing plants. A brief smile flickered across his face. "Have you ever participated in a *toma*, an ayahuasca session?" he asked.

"Once," I replied, "in Peru. But I know I have much to learn about the use of the vision vine for curing purposes." A fleeting, Mona Lisa smile played across his face as he stubbed out his cigarette on the dirt floor and said, "Then I'll see you at the ceremony tonight." And with that, he wandered off.

The session was held at a small tribal meetinghouse constructed at the edge of the village. I was crestfallen—the poured concrete floor, cinderblock walls, and corrugated aluminum roof seemed the very antithesis of rain forest culture. Where was the traditional *maloca*, the fantastic elongated conical roundhouse that was supposed to be the characteristic indigenous dwelling of the northwest Amazon? I asked a local Ingano fellow who wandered past. "The ayahuasca journey only begins there," he said, pointing with his chin at the structure. "But you will depart very quickly and travel very far away." He smiled and walked on.

The light of the moon on that clear evening was strong enough to illuminate enormous sandstone boulders that marked the edge of a small river running a few hundred meters to the west of the meetinghouse. On the other side of the water began the Andean foothills, home to the only pristine forest in the area. Surrounding the other sides of the meeting hall was nothing but depleted cattle pastures that had harbored magnificent rain forest until a few decades before.

The was an audible murmur from the other Indians as the shaman entered the hut. I marveled at the traditional *cushma*, the sky blue cotton tunic that covered him from shoulders to waist. Wrapped tightly around his thick biceps were dense strings of *shoroshoro* seeds that produced a hissing rattle as he walked. And around his neck was a magnificent necklace of jaguar teeth, the symbol of the shaman in many Amazonian tribes. It was only after admiring the medicine man's finery that I was startled to recognize him as the fellow with whom I had been chatting earlier that afternoon. In his ceremonial garb he looked every inch the great shaman, and I wondered how I could have ever thought otherwise.

The shaman took his seat on a low bench at one end of the hut while the rest of us sat in a circle on the dirt floor at his feet. A chilly breeze blew in from the Andean slopes and I shivered as much from anticipation as from the cold. The night was alive with jungle sounds: crickets buzzed and chirped, frogs croaked and trilled, nightjars cooed and whooped. Howler monkeys hooted briefly, indicating that rain would fall the next day.

The shaman dipped a calabash into an earthen pot between his feet. Holding it high over his head with both hands, he mumbled a few incantations before drinking the ayahuasca in a single draught. Wiping his mouth clean with the back of his hand, he refilled the container from the pot, repeated the incantation, and passed it to me.

I looked down at the cup and saw it filled to the brim with a thick reddish brown liquid. I tried to knock it back in one swallow as I had seen the shaman do. The dreadful bitterness of the potion, however, caught me by surprise and I struggled to keep from retching. The Indian seated on the other side of the shaman noted my distress and passed me a cup of *aguardiente,* a fiery sugar cane brandy whose sweet anise aftertaste erased the disagreeable brackishness of the ayahuasca. I sat and watched the shaman slowly repeat the procedure with everyone in the circle.

All seemed quiet and peaceful until the shaman picked up a handful of *wai-rah sacha* leaves and began to shake them in a fanning motion. The leaves produced a whistling sound not unlike a high wind rushing through the rain forest canopy before a heavy thunderstorm: *shhhhhh-shhhhhh.* He shook it in a slow, rhythmic pattern that proved hypnotic, and I felt as if my brain waves were being organized in a fixed laserlike pattern under his control. My body began to relax, and I lay back onto a blanket I had brought to ward off the cold. Glancing around, I noticed that everyone else had also reclined, as if the shaman had willed us to do so. Only the medicine man remained seated upright, and he began a mesmerizing chant: *Hey-yah-hey! Hey-yah-hey!*

What seems simple in retrospect was emotionally enrapturing at the time. And the shaking of the leaves added a layer of complexity and fascination that reverberated through my brain from the right front lobe to the rear left lobe to the rear right lobe to the front left lobe, and back again. By now the shaman seemed master of time, space, and my entire being.

I drifted off into a gentle trance. I felt myself lying in a tucum palm fiber hammock as comfortable as a giant feather bed. I was floating as in a dream. Looking up, I could see a beautiful blue tropical sky with only a few wisps of clouds above me. The hammock was slung between two towering columnar *epena* trees with a dark Amazonian lake below me. At the far edge of the lake I could make out the tiny figure of the shaman in this blue tunic continuing his chant. By the peaceful look on his face that I could just make out at this distance, I could tell that he was deep into his own ayahuasca visions. As I floated there with my hands propped comfortably behind my head, I peacefully reviewed scenes from my life that reenacted themselves for my analysis. Aside from a few mild waves of nausea, all seemed peaceful and calm; I was at one with the cosmos.

Soon the shaman ceased his chant, and I opened my eyes to find myself seated at his feet once more. He refilled the calabash, prayed over it, and drank it down. Repeating the first two steps, he then passed the container to me. I drained it but it didn't sit right in my stomach. I tried to ignore the volcanic nausea welling up inside. I promised myself that I would lie back down as soon as everyone had had their turn and began to feel a bit better by focusing all my attention on the shaman. I knew that he was able to feel my gaze, and he turned to me. As he did so, the beaded bracelets on his biceps produced the sound of rushing water and turned into tiny glowing diamonds that all but obscured my field of vision. As the diamonds dissipated, I could see that the shaman was staring at me with a look that combined equal parts power, disdain, humor, and kindness. I stared at his black pupils growing larger and larger, finally combining into one giant black vortex into which I was sucked. I was underwater now in waters as pitch-black as the Rio Negro. Huge black caimans and anacondas swarmed in the river, menacing me with their size and demeanor, though not attacking me directly. Running out of air, and afraid of the creatures that surrounded me in this aquatic realm, I swam desperately.

I broke the surface and crawled on all fours onto a white sandy beach along the riverbank. Having been underwater too long, I became sick, vomiting and vomiting. I was unable to stop; the life began ebbing from my body. I could not regain my feet and sank face down into the sand, rising up enough only to retch over to the side. I began weeping and begging for help as I continued to fade. Pain racked my body and my head felt as if it had exploded. I tried fighting for my life but no longer had the strength. I had managed to crawl up the riverbank toward the jungle but only made it far enough to pass out in the grass at the edge of the forest. I lay face down. I died.

I don't know how long I lay in the grass, inert, comatose, inanimate. But I could hear something in the back of my head. The shaman continued to chant, deep in the forest in front of me. With a Herculean effort, I managed to raise myself on all fours. I began weeping again because I did not have the strength to go to him. As I sat mired in this predicament, I was frightened by a deep guttural grunt in the jungle in front of me. A jaguar! Now I was weak *and* terrified. But a most extraordinary thing happened: the great cat's roar caused a wave of nausea to well up inside me and I puked as I never had before. Horrible things poured out of me: purple frogs and bloodred snakes and phosphorescent orange scorpions. I thought I was dying a second death, yet when it stopped I felt a bit stronger. So close was the jaguar that I could smell him, yet I was no longer afraid. I stumbled a bit as I followed him into the jungle; I knew that he was leading me toward the shaman. Tripping over roots, I tried to keep pace with the great cat. I momentarily worried about snakes until I realized that nothing could be worse than what I was enduring.

Falling to my knees, I looked up to see the shaman standing over me. He began a peculiar chant that made my head hurt even more until he pressed his palms against my temples and started to squeeze. As he twisted my neck to the right I felt my vertebrae pop; the pain began to abate, ever so slightly. He seated me on a tree trunk and began to dance around me. Taking a swig of an herbal tea, he circled me, spitting the aromatic liquid at me in a cold spray at each of the four cardinal points of the compass. The pain and confusion that racked my body began to subside as he massaged my arms and neck. The sun had started to rise in the east. He sang and rubbed my upper body with leaves, pausing every now and again to cast off some invisible film he seemed to be scraping off me. I managed to croak out a question: "Why did you do this to me?"

He gave a cryptic, Cheshire cat smile and replied: "You have had a glimpse of our world. You have been purged, cleaned, healed. You will never again fear death as you have now died and been reborn."

In a classic treatise on ayahuasca (1979), R. E. Schultes wrote:

> There is a magic intoxicant in northwesternmost South America which the Indians believe can free the soul from corporeal confinement, allowing it to wander free and return to the body at will. The soul, thus untrammeled, liberates its owner from the everyday life and introduces him to wondrous realms of what he considers reality and permits him to communicate with his ancestors. The Kechua term for this inebriating drink—ayahuasca ("vine of the soul")—refers to this freeing of the spirit. The plants involved are truly plants of the gods, for their powers are laid to supernatural forces residing in their tissues, and they were the divine gifts to the earliest Indians on earth. The drink employed for prophecy, divination, sorcery, and medical purposes, is so deeply rooted in native mythology and philosophy that there can be no doubt of its great age as part of aboriginal life.

In the northwest Amazon, ayahuasca represents an essential component of most—if not all—shamanic healing ceremonies. Yet there are aspects of these shamanic practices that are used by other cultures around the world, only some of which employ psychotropic plants in their healing rituals. According to Dr. Piers Vitebsky, an authority on Eurasian shamanism, the word "shaman" comes from the language of the Evenk peoples, reindeer herders in Siberia. To the Evenk, a shaman is a person who can "will his or her spirit to leave the body and journey to upper or lower world." Common elements unite the shamanic tradition found on every continent except Antarctica.

Curing disease, preventing famine, controlling the weather, entering trances, fighting evil spirits sent by malevolent shamans of other tribes, traveling up to the spirit world, or conveying souls to the underworld are common denominators among most practitioners of what we consider shamanism. In most groups, the shaman serves as the only tribal member who fully comprehends both the "real" world and the "spirit" world and is therefore responsible for maintaining the balance between the two.

Within the context of the source culture, shamanism is often considered a profoundly holy profession. Unlike in much of the industrialized world, in which healing is essentially divorced from spirituality, the shaman also functions as the priest-rabbi, which greatly augments his or her ability to heal. As Western science finally begins to study and appreciate the therapeutic benefits of spirituality, the practice and effectiveness of shamanism becomes not only more comprehensible but also more appreciated.

An integral component of shamanistic healing is what has been called "the placebo effect." Many leaders of the Western medical establishment came of age during the antibiotic revolution, the single greatest therapeutic advance of the mid-twentieth century. However, the development of these drugs also led several generations of physicians to equate (to a large degree) chemistry and healing. Spirituality (its nature and its role in healing) was part of few (if any) medical school curricula. The placebo effect, in which patients recovered because they believed they would, was not in and of itself shunned, but more often noted with bemusement rather than harnessed and put to work.

Shamans, on the other hand, are masters of the placebo effect. Much has been made of the shamanic practice of sucking the "evil darts" (or other foreign substances) out of the patient's body by the healer. References in the literature often refer to it as trickery or sleight of hand, usually in a condescending way. Two aspects, however, are overlooked. First, it often provides the patient some relief, convincing them that they are on the road to recovery and creating a mind-set that facilitates healing. Second, therapeutic compounds, usually in the form of plants, are also employed because the shaman is customarily a master botanist. The shaman's genius as a healer stems from his (or her) ability to combine the spiritual (sucking out evil darts, communing with the forces of nature, etc.) with the chemical (the plants, insects, etc.)

Chief Pierce of Flat Iron, an Oglala Sioux, explained the inextricable link between the holy and the botanical almost a century ago: "From Wakan-Tanka, the Great Mystery, comes all power. . . . Man knows that all healing plants are given by Wakan-Tanka: therefore they are holy. . . . The Great Mystery gave to men all things for their food, their clothing, their welfare. And to man he gave also the knowledge how to use these gifts . . . how to find the holy healing plants."

The sophisticated botanical knowledge of these "uneducated" shamans astonishes Western researchers. In the rain forest, these healers can sometimes identify almost every single species of tree merely by the smell, appearance, or feel of the bark, a feat no university-trained botanist can accomplish. And their knowledge of the ecology of these plants—when they fruit, when they flower, what pollinates them, what disperses the seeds, what preys on them, what type of soil they prefer—is no less impressive. As nature continues to provide us with a cornucopia of new medicines, these shamans (in the rain forest and elsewhere) will prove to be the ultimate sources of knowledge about which species offer therapeutic promise and how they might best be employed.

Almost every plant species that has been put to use by Western medicine was originally discovered and utilized by indigenous cultures. Despite the fact that a single shaman may know and employ over a hundred species for medicinal purposes, or that a single tribe (which may have several shamans) may know and utilize several hundred species for medical purposes, few of the world's remaining tribal peoples have been the subject of comprehensive ethnobotanical/ethnomedical studies. Yet the more we study, the more we learn how little we know about how much they know.

Ayahuasca, the vision vine, represents a classic example. The early accounts of ayahuasca focused on a single species of vine (*Banisteriopsis caapi*). Subsequent research has revealed that other plants added to the mixture determine the actual type, intensity, and duration of the hallucinations—proving the sophistication of these shamans as both botanists and chemists. For example, leaves of a species of the *Psychotria* shrub of the coffee family are often added to the ayahuasca mixture. These leaves contain chemicals called tryptamines that induce hallucinations. The compounds, however, are inactive when taken orally unless activated by the presence of another type of chemical known as monoamine oxidase inhibitors. The psychotropic compounds in the ayahuasca vine not only induce hallucinations but also function as monoamine oxidase inhibitors. The result: a brew much more potent than one prepared from either species.

Furthermore, the shamans often have the remarkable ability to distinguish between, describe, and make use of distinct healing and/or chemical properties of different parts of the same plant. A shaman, for example, will note that bark from the upper stem of the ayahuasca vine may cause visions of jaguars, while the root bark results in scenes of anacondas. Schultes wrote:

> Among the Tukano of the Colombian Vaupes, for example, six "kinds" of Ayahuasca or Kahi are recognized. . . . *Kahi riama*, the strongest, produces auditory hallucinations and announces future events. It is said to cause death if improperly employed. The second strongest, *Mene-kahi-ma*, reputedly causes visions of green snakes. . . . These two "kinds" may not belong to Ban-

isteriopsis or even to the family Malpighiaceae. The third in strength is called *Suana-kahi-ma* ("Kahi of the red jaguar"), producing visions in red. *Kahi-vai Bucura-rijoma* ("Kahi of the monkey head") causes monkeys to hallucinate and howl. . . . All of these "kinds" are referable probably to *Banisteriopsis caapi* [e.g., what to Western botanists is all the same species].

Hallucinogens, while an integral part of shamanic healing practices in the western Amazon, still represent only a very small portion of plants employed for therapeutic purposes. As we have seen before, natural products employed for a particular purpose in one culture may offer promise of a different use in our own culture. In the case of ayahuasca, for example, Western-trained physicians in both Brazil and Peru are using the vine as an experimental treatment for chronic alcoholism and crack addiction, with promising results.

An example of using one therapeutic plant for different purposes in a different culture comes to us from the tropical forests of American Samoa in the South Pacific, where the herbal healers—the *taulasea*—are primarily women. These herbalists know 200 species of plants and recognize 180 types of diseases. Ethnobotanist Dr. Paul Cox of the National Tropical Botanical Garden had been working with this culture for over a decade when, in 1984, a *taulasea* named Epenesa Mauigoa showed him an herbal treatment for acute hepatitis prepared from the inner bark of a local species of rubber tree. Cox was particularly intrigued when she insisted that only one "variety" of the tree could be employed when, in Western botanical terms, both varieties were the same species. Investigation of the plant in the laboratories of the National Cancer Institute outside Washington, D.C., yielded a new molecule that the scientists named prostratin. This compound belongs to a class of chemicals known as phorbols, many of which cause tumors in the human body. Intriguingly, however, prostratin not only inhibited the formation of tumors but, in the test tube, prevented cells from becoming infected by the HIV-1 virus and extended the life of infected cells! Of course, it is a long way from the jungle to the laboratory and, in some ways, an even longer trail from the test tube to the pharmacy. Nonetheless, research on prostratin continues. And it is precisely these finds that validate indigenous wisdom in Western eyes, leading to pharmaceutical companies' increased interest in shamanic wisdom.

Scientists continue to be astonished at the breadth and depth of indigenous wisdom. Ethnobotanists at the New York Botanical Garden recently conducted a classic comparative study of indigenous ethnobotanical sagacity in the Amazon Basin. Working with the Chacobo tribe in Bolivia, Dr. Brian Boom found they used 95 percent of the local tree species. His colleague Dr. Bill Balee learned that the Tembe peoples of Brazil employed 61.3 percent of local trees while the Ka'apoor tribe used 76.8 percent.

The effectiveness of this wisdom is being validated in the laboratory. Dr. Bernard Ortiz de Montellano of Wayne State University sifted through accounts of the ethnomedicine of the Aztec peoples of ancient Mexico and was able to identify 118 plants that they employed as medicines. When he subjected them to laboratory examination, he found that almost 85 percent were at least somewhat efficacious, strikingly similar to data gathered by Paul Cox and his colleagues in Polynesia. The joint Swedish-American research team tested the Samoan medicinal plants in the laboratory. The results: 86 percent demonstrated significant pharmacological activity.

Of course, new mechanisms must be developed to protect the intellectual property rights of these local peoples and local governments: fortunately, the colonial/neocolonial model of "Let's take what we need of local plants and wisdom and cart it off to the marketplace" is completely unacceptable as we enter the twenty-first century. New economic models and legal frameworks are being devised and put in place to share benefits from these new discoveries and avoid the "rape and run" approach to commercializing natural resources that characterized much of human history.

Nonetheless, an enormous body of shamanic knowledge remains untested (or untestable) in the laboratory because we cannot (or have not yet been able to) understand it outside of the context of indigenous culture. The Tirio Indians of the northeast Amazon, for example, employ a series of plants to treat ailments that (they claim) are caused by the breaking of hunting taboos. One ancient medicine man showed me a plant that he explained was "boiled into a tea and given to an infant who was crying at night because he couldn't sleep because his father had killed a giant anteater." Another species was used for the same purpose, except that the child suffered insomnia because the father had killed a tapir. Most Westerners would regard these ailments as imaginary. A much more effective utilitarian approach, instead of dismissing this seemingly incomprehensible claim, would be to investigate whether the plant potion contained compounds that might serve as the basis for a safe, effective, nonaddictive sleeping pill—a potion that Western medicine has been unable to devise.

In our culture, we have been taught that our system of medicine (and other things!) is the most advanced, the most successful, the most sophisticated, and so on—a valid statement, in many regards. This "lesson," however, often results in a cultural arrogance that underestimates or even denigrates other systems, either because they seem "primitive" and/or because we don't understand what they are trying to tell or teach us. In his brilliant book *Witch-doctors and Psychiatrists,* Dr. E. Fuller Torrey wrote: "A psychiatrist who tells an illiterate African that his phobia is related to fear of failure and a witch doctor who tells an American tourist that his phobia is related to possession by an ancestral spirit will be met by equally blank stares."

Our culture teaches us to "cut to the chase," to get that one plant or (better yet) one molecule that is responsible for the shaman's cure—and you can spare us the magic rattle and the sacred smoke, thank you very much. Some of these cures only work within their cultural context, be it a treatment for possession by an ancestral spirit, a cure that involves ceremony, ritual, and healing plants, or a mundane remedy that simply requires rubbing a few crushed leaves on the afflicted area. Clearly, some of these treatments harness powerful chemicals that can be used effectively far from their site of origin and within a Western (or other) clinical context.

The Western tendency to adopt a reductionist approach is not just an interest in getting to the basic chemistry (preferably a single molecule that is responsible for the therapeutic effect) or merely a question of being in a hurry—it is also a question of safety and economics. It has proven difficult, if not impossible, to patent a complex plant extract that may contain a multitude of chemicals, even if proven safe and effective. Still, our cultural propensity to reduce everything to the simplest common denominator can cause us to underestimate or even deny the shaman's healing wisdom. A recent example: two ethnobotanists were intrigued by a West African medicine man who appeared to have an extremely potent potion for reducing blood-sugar levels in diabetic patients. They asked whether he might be willing to provide them with the plants he used so they could take them back to the United States for testing. The shaman readily agreed and gave the scientists three different plants. In the lab, they tested species A, which had no effect; they tried species B, which had no effect. They tested species C, still with no positive results. Finally, they boiled them all together and analyzed the resulting potion. Nothing! A year later, back in Africa, they returned to the medicine man. "Your potion doesn't seem to work," said one of the ethnobotanists to the witch doctor.

"What do you mean?" he replied. "You saw me give it to my patients, and measured their blood-sugar levels with your instruments. You yourself told me that the blood-sugar level went down. How could you now claim it doesn't work?"

The ethnobotanists then asked the medicine man if he would be willing to prepare a batch of the potion they could then take with them. He agreed. The shaman boiled water in a big aluminum pot over a wood fire. He added the first plant species, then the second, then the third. Just as he was preparing to take the pot off the fire, he reached into a wet muslin sack, extracted a crab, and dropped it in the pot.

"What is that?" asked one of the ethnobotanists.

"What does it look like?" replied the shaman. "It is a crab!"

"Yeah, I know," responded the scientist. "But why did you add it to the pot? You didn't tell us that was part of the recipe."

The shaman smiled. "Look," he said, "you asked me if I would give you the plants used to make the potion. I did!"

The scientists took the potion back to the United States, found it to be effective at lowering blood sugar, and it is currently being investigated in the lab.

Of course, a shaman's healing wizardry does not necessarily entail the use of nature's chemistry. Dr. Charles Limbach, an American physician with extensive experience in Latin America, recently related an intriguing encounter. A friend of his, also a physician, had returned from a sojourn in the Oriente, the Amazonian territory of eastern Ecuador:

My friend was visiting a missionary acquaintance who was working with the Shuar people, also called the Jivaro, who were once renowned for their then common practice of removing and then shrinking the heads of their enemies. He was sitting on the porch of the missionary's house and chatting with his fellow American and an elderly Shuar who had a reputation as a powerful shaman. While they were conversing, another Shuar arrived and asked the missionary for help with a botfly larva (through a complicated process, botfly eggs enter the human body and hatch into larvae which feed on human flesh. The standard western treatment is to cut them out with a scalpel). The missionary, who had received some medical training, ducked into the house and came back out with alcohol, cotton swabs, a bandage, and a scalpel. The Shuar shaman asked what he planned to do with all that equipment. The American replied that he would cut out the larva. The shaman smiled, and said he would handle it. He sat the patient in a hammock, leaned over the arm with the botfly and began to sing. Within minutes, the botfly larva emerged from the man's arm, fell onto the floor of the porch, and the shaman crushed it beneath his bare foot.

Neither Limbach nor his colleague was able to explain the incident. Had the shaman sung at a particular frequency maddening to the insect, as opera singers are able to hit a note that can shatter glass? Or did the shaman surreptitiously exhale tobacco smoke into the larva's breathing hole, causing it to crawl out in search of air? In some ways, this situation is analogous to the use of aspirin for most of the past century: even though we didn't fully understand how it functioned in the human body until relatively recently, we nonetheless used the drug because it was safe, effective, and painless.

The extraordinary antiquity of shamanistic practices is well documented. Southern France has long been famous for a series of caves, the walls of which are covered with the oldest known art of human origin. Several years ago, the most ancient of all was discovered not far from other subterranean caverns that had been known and studied for over a century. This cave, christened Chauvet, contained art that was noticeably similar to that found in the earlier discoveries, with portrayals of large mammals like the cave bear and woolly rhinoceros that flourished in Europe at that time. On a hanging rock near the entrance, however, is a striking portrait of a composite creature, the bottom half of which is a human, the upper half a bison. Here, in the earliest known example of human art ever discovered, we see the portrait of the shaman.

Chauvet Cave has been dated at well over thirty thousand years old, which means that this art was created twenty-five thousand years before the more familiar paintings and sculpture of "ancient" Egypt. Similar half-man half-beast motifs are found in many caverns painted and carved in the distant past. The best known and most thoroughly studied of the caves is at Lascaux; a man in a bird mask lies next to a staff with a bird on the end of it. The bird that—unlike most humans—can soar over the forest and through the heavens represents the symbol of the shaman in many cultures.

Joseph Campbell suggested that this particular figure lies "rapt in a shamanistic trance" and that "in that remote period of our species the arts of the wizard, shaman, or magician were already well developed."

The Trois Frères sanctuary dates from fourteen thousand years ago and harbors what is probably the most famous prehistoric painting of a shaman: the Dancing Sorcerer. The magnificent portrait features a male creature composed of the parts of many different animals. It has antlers on its head, yet dances on its hind legs in a clearly human manner. Adding further credence that this is a human rather than an animal is the headdress of caribou antlers worn in sacred dances by shamans of Arctic and subarctic tribes, much as Indian medicine men on the Great Plains wore headdresses of buffalo horns.

The antiquity of healing-plant knowledge is assumed to be equally great. A Neanderthal grave at Shanidar in Iraq, near the Iran border, held seven species of plants carefully buried around the corpse. People living in the region today use five of those seven species for medicinal purposes. At Monte Verde in southern Chile, recently concluded to be the site of the earliest known habitation in South America, researchers found what had been gardens of medicinal plants. A ubiquitous species was an evergreen shrub known locally as *boldo,* and widely used as a diuretic, a laxative, and a treatment for liver problems. Laboratory research has proven that this plant is an effective diuretic; investigations in Germany have led to its official approval for the treatment of stomach and intestinal cramps as well as dyspepsia.

The question then arises as to the source of ethnomedical wisdom: simply stated, how did the shamans learn which plants had healing properties? Trial and error undoubtedly played a central role. But in a place like the Amazon, with eighty thousand species of flowering plants (not to mention tens of millions of other organisms), how would the healers know not only which plant to employ but which part of the plant to use? And at what dosage? How did the shaman learn at which phase of the moon these plants should be collected? Even more curious is how they devised such clever recipes that sometimes consist of over twenty components. In the instance of the diabetes case history presented in the introduction, the shaman made the potion from four plants. What would be the odds of recreating that potion using the correct dosage, species, and particular plant parts from a forest of eighty thousand species if we tried to do it based on random collections, which has been the major approach used by most pharmaceutical companies up to the present date?

One key as to how the shamans and others have found and utilized species with therapeutic compounds is the taste test. The concept of "bitter" exists in most cultures, and bitterness often indicates the presence of alkaloids, which represent the single most important chemical components of modern medicine. Quinine and ayahuasca are some of the bitterest substances known.

Yet another clue for the shamans also serves as a lead for Western scientists like David Newman or William Fenical, who look for new medicines from marine organisms: color equals chemistry. If a plant (particularly a tree sap) has a peculiar color, it may well contain interesting chemicals. The clear red sap of the *Virola* tree led shamans of the Yanomami people of Venezuela to develop it into a powerful hallucinogenic snuff, just as the brilliant orange sap of the *Vismia* bush of Suriname led the Tirio shamans to use it as an effective treatment for fungal infections of the skin. The milky red sap of the *Croton* tree led Shuar shamans to employ it as a safe and effective agent for healing wounds.

Another key is the so-called doctrine of signatures. Simply stated, if a plant (or plant part) looks like something, it is somehow good for that something. In other words, because a walnut looks like a brain, it must be good for diseases afflicting the brain (a common belief in medieval Europe). As ludicrous as it sounds, the doctrine has yielded at least one medicinal compound in wide use until recently. The Vedas of ancient India were written about four thousand years ago and included a remedy for snakebite from the snakeroot plant, so named because the twisted roots resembled squirming serpents. Tested in the laboratory in the 1950s, it was found ineffective for countering the toxic effects of the snake venom. One of the problems associated with snakebite, however, is that the trauma of being bitten causes the heart to beat faster, thus pumping the poison throughout the system. What the alkaloid in snakeroot does do is slow down the heartbeat and, because of this, was developed into one of the first effective tranquilizers used by Western medicine.

Once again, this demonstrates why we should not reject ideas gleaned from other medical systems without first investigating them. The Aztecs valued a Mexican species of magnolia with a heart-shaped fruit as a treatment for cardiac problems. Recent investigations in the lab have found that this fruit contains compounds with a digitalis-like activity.

The most intriguing source of ideas for which plants can be utilized medicinally is perhaps the most difficult concept for Westerners to accept: a shaman's dreams. After a ten-year hiatus, in 1995 I returned to the village of Tepoe in Suriname while searching for diabetes treatments and sought out the great shaman Mahshewah. The old healer, though he appeared pleased at my return, said that he was unable to help me. "I'm sorry," he said, "but I don't recall ever seeing that disease so I can't tell you what plant might be useful for treating it."

Six days later, Mahshewah summoned me to his hut, where he related a most interesting occurrence: "This afternoon I was sleeping in my hammock and I had a dream. And in this dream I saw a tree, and the bark of this tree may help to treat this disease that you said is killing your people. If you canoe down the river for about an hour and a half, you will find a trail on the west bank. If you walk up this trail for about an hour, you will find an enormous tree with yellowish peeling bark. That is the species whose bark may help your people."

I followed his directions down the river and found the trail. I followed his directions up the trail and found the tree. Mahshewah's legs have been paralyzed since he was born. When I asked the other Indians if the old medicine man had ever been up that trail, they told me unequivocally that he had not. How does one explain this through the prism of Western science? I gathered a few scrapings of the bark because my guide said it was a rare and sacred tree that could not be collected in bulk. We still do not know if it might prove efficacious in treating the disease.

The question as to whether something useful can be "discovered" through dreams is one that many people in our society would be inclined to answer negatively. Yet how many remember the discovery of the structure of benzene? Friedrich August Kekulé von Stradowitz, one of the greatest chemists of nineteenth-century Europe, simply could not figure out the structure of the molecule of this enormously important industrial solvent. Quitting in frustration, he decided to turn in for the night and tackle the problem again in the morning. Soon he was dreaming and in his dream he saw several snakes. One of the reptiles began chasing another and then the others joined in, forming a circle. Kekulé woke up with the solution to the problem: benzene is a ring! When British scientists dream the answer to perplexing problems, they may become famous, rich, well-respected, and sometimes offered a knighthood. But when Amazonian shamans do it, we dismiss it as "unscientific."

Mother Nature herself is a great teacher. In the words of the gifted natural history writer Sy Montgomery: "In other, older cultures than our own, in which people live closer to the earth, humans do not look down on animals from an imaginary pinnacle. Life is not divided between animals and people, nonhuman and human: life is a continuum, interactive, interdependent. Humans and animals are considered companions and coplayers in the drama of life. Animals' lives, their motives and thoughts and feelings, deserve human attention and respect; dismissing their importance is a grave error."

Characteristic among indigenous cultures of North America was the famous "vision quest," in which a young man (often an apprentice shaman) would go into the wilderness to pray and fast, fast and pray. After several days, he would be visited by visions, often in the form of an animal that would, in the words of the great Inuit shaman Igjugarjuk, "open the mind of a man to all that is hidden to others." As a result of this vision quest, the boy often ended up with a totemic spirit, an animal that served as his personal symbol or protector. The shaman may conclude the process with "animal familiars" or "power animals"—an animal or animals that help him learn and heal. So close is the identification with the animal that the shaman may be perceived as part animal, an essential component of sacred tribal dances around the world and the ancient cave paintings from Europe. In some cultures, the shamans believe that they actually become the animals, as do the Tirio shamans in the northeast Amazon, who claim the ability to turn into jaguars and roam the jungle at night. Among many tribes, the shaman becomes a bird, omniscient by virtue of his or her ability to look down from above and see things invisible to all others. In the case of the Navajo, as we saw in the last chapter, the bear is the medicinal plant master who taught the Indians about *Ligusticum* and all other healing plants.

The realization that much of shamanic knowledge is based on animals' use of plants is relatively new to Western scientific thought. As we saw in the previous chapter, many healing plants employed by tribespeople have probably been learned from local animals. The legends of these cultures often feature sagas explaining how people first learned of useful plants (agricultural and medicinal) from forest creatures. In these cases, animals are, perhaps both metaphorically and literally, the bringers of wisdom.

Joseph Campbell suggested that true shamanism is the religion of the original hunting societies; with the advent of agriculture, cultures became more communally oriented and their religious beliefs changed. While this argument is somewhat hypothetical, what is more certain is that the manifestations of shamanistic religion have been seen as a threat by other organized religions, particularly Christianity, which saw itself in direct competition with belief systems that offered extraordinary experiences to the adherents: "The white goes into his church and talks about Jesus; the Indian walks into his teepee and talks to Jesus," wrote one anthropologist, describing peyote rituals among Native American peoples. But consider this passage from the Book of Job: "But ask now the beasts, and they shall teach thee; and the fowls of the air, and they shall teach thee."

The supreme irony of our suppression of, or disregard for, shamanic religions or other medical practices that rely on natural products is not only the extraordinary therapeutic gifts they have already provided us, but our undeniable need for more of these healing potions to treat "incurable" diseases. The witches of medieval Europe, burned at the stake for their heretical beliefs, were the shamans and/or herbalists of their day. It was their ethnopharmacopeia that gave us aspirin and digitalis. And if we had paid closer attention to their custom of applying moldy bread to wounds, we might have "discovered" penicillin several centuries earlier than Alexander Fleming's research in the 1920s.

A similar situation transpired in our own country. We have all heard about how Squanto and his fellow Indians taught the Pilgrims how to farm the land, but what did the settlers use for medicine? Native American medicinal plants cured the Pilgrims' ailments just as Native American crops filled the European bellies. And prior to the arrival of these Europeans, some of the original Americans had learned that mold could hasten the healing of wounds and local foxglove could treat certain heart problems. Native American healers independently invented syringes and enemas, developed a local anesthetic, and conducted head surgery. Every medicinal plant valued by the settlers was taught to them by local tribespeople. Some of these species entered into commercial, over-the-counter drugs: the yellow color of Murine eyedrops was until recently due to alkaloids extracted from the goldenseal herb. Others, like cascara sagrada (a common ingredient in many laxatives), are sold in many pharmacies. And new medicines are still being developed from plants originally employed by Native Americans: extracts of American bloodroot now serve as an antiplaque agent in toothpastes.

Even some of the most troublesome medical problems are being treated by ancient Indian medicines. Benign prostate enlargement (BPH) afflicts tens of thousands of American men. The fruits of the saw palmetto, a scrubby palm from the southeastern United States, have proven extremely effective at reducing the symptoms: as effective, it has been claimed, as a medicine marketed by Merck.

·   ·   ·

Neither nature nor the shaman has all the answers to the ills that plague us, but both have some—I would say many—of these answers. Urgently needed is an approach that is more humble, more spiritual, more environmental, and more open-minded. The great anthropologist Weston LaBarre, who collaborated with R. E. Schultes on his early peyote research, wrote of the South American Indian:

> As scientists we cannot afford the luxury of an ethnocentric snobbery which assumes *a priori* that primitive cultures have nothing whatsoever to contribute to civilization. Our civilization is, in fact, a compendium of such borrowings, and it is a demonstrable error to believe that contacts of "higher" and "lower" cultures show benefits flowing exclusively in one direction. Indeed, a good case could probably be made that in the long run it is the "higher" culture which benefits the more through being enriched, while the "lower" culture not uncommonly disappears entirely as a result of the contact.

Twenty years ago, I stumbled across the most moving account of this ongoing tragedy that I have ever seen—and it was all because of an earache.

A common and painful ailment suffered by researchers working in the rain forest is fungal infection of the ear. The hot and wet environment of the tropics turns eardrums into petri dishes ripe for the cultivation of fungal invaders. When I began working in the Amazon in the late 1970s, I developed these infections on such a regular basis that before departing I would schedule appointments to have my ears examined at the university clinic upon my return to the States. I quickly learned that if I mentioned my occupation to the physician on duty, she or he would often tell me at great length that ethnobotany was what they really wanted to do with their careers but that they had student loans, a mortgage, a family, and so on, which was why they had been unable to pursue this dream.

I vividly remember going into the clinic with a terrible earache after an expedition to the jungles of southern Venezuela. After examining my ear, attending physician Dr. Jonathan Strongin asked if

I had any idea where I might have picked up such a peculiar fungus. "Sure," I replied, "I've just returned from South America."

He asked what I had been doing south of the border, and I gave a distinctly noncommittal reply. He said, "You know, I lived with Indians in the Peruvian Amazon for several years while I was doing my Ph.D. in anthropology, which is how I became interested in healing."

Intrigued, I made a mental note of his name, looked up his dissertation, and found one of the most poignant statements ever recorded on the inextricable interrelationship between people, plants, healing, and belief:

> Since the time of their initial contact, the missionaries have openly discouraged the [shamans], viewing them as Anti-Christs. . . . [Another anthropologist reported] that in the Shimaa region there was a powerful [shaman] who had to abandon his craft because he felt he no longer had the support of the Machiguenga people in his area. This shaman used ayahuasca to take the form of a bird to travel far and wide at a great height to discern the cause of illness. However, he felt that because the missionaries had so successfully eroded the traditional faith of his people, he could no longer continue to cure. For without the faith of the population, while in the avian form he would not be able to return to his body and [would] crash in the forest far from home . . .

The Sugar Sickness

Just a little over ten months after I had watched the Sikiyana shaman treat the Tirio woman for diabetes, I returned to the little village in the northeast Amazon. I had been collecting plants nearby, and wished to take advantage of this opportunity to see how the patient had fared under the care of the medicine man.

After a brief palaver with the chief, who welcomed me back and granted me permission to spend a week in the village, I headed for the hut of the woman who had been dying of diabetes. A seven-year-old boy stood in front of the hut, shooting tiny arrows at passing lizards with his toy bow.

"*Anpo nai emama?*" I asked. "Where's your mother?"

"*Wakin shenpo, meinjare tebita,*" he replied. "She's not here. She's working in the family garden today."

That she was able to work I took as a favorable sign.

I then went in search of the Sikiyana shaman, but he was out hunting and was not expected back until after sunset. Shouldering my backpack, which I had left with the chief, I headed for an old hut near the river's edge where I had stayed during my previous visit.

Later that afternoon, after a brief but powerful thundershower had swept through and cooled the torpid air, I was lying in my hammock and gazing out over the river as a dugout canoe loaded to the gunwales with women, dogs, and a mountain of cassava roots came drifting past my hut. Landing just upriver, they began to off-load the cassava. Before I could even ponder the question of whether to offer some assistance, I saw who I was looking for and went racing down the riverbank.

Before me stood the diabetic, hunched over forward with what must have been close to a hundred pounds of cassava tied into her backpack, preparing to climb up to the village. A bit shocked by having a white man in gym shorts and sandals accost her, she unshouldered the backpack and stood up straight to get a better look at me.

I was momentarily speechless. When I had arrived during my previous visit, she had been dying. The shaman had given her the medicine, and she had begun to recover by the time of my departure. But I could not believe what I was now seeing: she appeared to be the personification of good health. Though dirty and sweaty from working in the garden, her eyes were so clear and bright that they sparkled. Her skin was a lustrous walnut-brown and she gave me a dazzling smile. Flustered, I looked down. Her bare feet showed no evidence of the ugly diabetic sores that had festered between her toes on my last visit.

"Re-Remember me?" I asked, out of breath and flustered after having lost all semblance of dignity by running up to her.

"Yes," she replied. "What is it you want?" She clearly had more important tasks than making small talk with a visitor, even one she had met before.

I, on the other hand, had many questions. How was she feeling? How was she doing? How long had she been working? Was she still taking the medicine?

Re-hoisting the backpack, she answered my queries as she climbed the riverbank, her bare feet skillfully planted in the slippery mud, as I floundered behind her in my sandals. I followed her to her hut as she answered my questions.

She felt fine, she told me, and had started working in her garden on a regular basis within weeks of my previous departure. No, she didn't take the medicine every day, only when the symptoms of the disease began to reappear, about once a month, at which point she had the shaman prepare the same potion. She would drink the medicine three times a day and the symptoms would disappear after a week.

By now, we had reached her thatched hut, and she made it clear the interview had ended. I thanked her for the information as she ducked inside.

On the fourth day, the shaman, who had been on a hunting expedition, reappeared. Having heard I'd been asking for him, he came looking for me before I knew that he had returned. We chatted a bit, and I told him how impressed I was with the status of the woman's health. He shot me a knowing smile. "She's not the only one, you know," he said. "Two other women with the same problem asked my help after you left. They weren't as bad off as the woman you saw, but the medicine was just as effective for them."

"Look," I said, "this disease is killing my people. It killed my grandmother, and many people in my country die from this sickness every year. Might it be possible to test it in my country? If we can make a medicine from it, you and your people will benefit as well. Please think it over, and let me know your decision."

The shaman gave me a cryptic smile.

The next night, I had a lengthy meeting with the shaman, the chief, and the village elders. We reached an agreement on compensation and established a contractual agreement that satisfied everyone.

I collected the plants, brought them back to the States, had them analyzed in the lab, and the results were negative.

I returned the following year, had the shaman prepare the actual potion, brought it back for testing, and the results were again negative. Meanwhile, the three women in the village, who had been certified as diabetics by a visiting physician, continued to enjoy robust health while taking the shaman's potion.

Puzzled and frustrated, I asked a chemist who had worked on the analysis if he could explain the discrepancy between what I was seeing in the field and what was happening (or not happening) in the laboratory. He noted that lab analysis often consists of an initial search for the "therapeutically active compounds"—the chemicals powerful enough to account for the action of the potion—and then the testing of each component separately. Shamanistic medicine often depends on synergy, how the chemical components of the herbs interact with each other, or how the shaman's practices—chanting, aromatherapy, or massage, in some cases—create a mental state that interacts with the plant chemicals.

When I asked the shaman, his reply was similar to that of the chemist. "You want to know which is the most important plant in the recipe, but that tells me you don't understand my medicine. I make the potion from four plants and *every plant in the potion contributes to the healing process.* Do you think I would waste my time seeking and adding useless plants to my medicine?" He mistook my innocence for impudence, and the research was at an impasse.

Meanwhile, diabetes continues to kill not only our people, but people around the world. More than 15 million Americans are diabetic, and approximately 175,000 die as a result of the disease each year. Nor is the suffering caused by diabetes restricted to fatalities: thousands will have to have feet amputated, more than 10,000 will go blind, and virtually all suffer greater risk of stroke and heart disease. Meanwhile, more than 125 million outside the United States suffer from diabetes. As the rest of the world adopts the worst aspects of the West—high-fat diets coupled with a sedentary lifestyle—the incidence of diabetes will increase sharply.

Diabetes, drug-resistant bacteria, intractable pain—all these causes of human suffering and death obligate us to search for new treatments and cures. Plants, ants, frogs, and the shaman's knowledge as to how best to use them offer potential solutions to some of the health problems that plague us. It would be foolish to assert that nature can cure every ailment, but it would be much more absurd to claim that all of Mother Nature's healing secrets have already been revealed. We still don't understand how this shaman's medicine is working: Is it "simply" the placebo effect? Is there some hidden ingredient that he refuses to reveal? Or is our desire to find the "magic bullet"—the single compound that would account for the potion's effectiveness—failing because the synergy of different compounds is what makes the medicine work? This represents but one example of how we were unable to decipher all of nature's mysteries during the twentieth century and are unlikely to do so during the next one, either. What we will be able to accomplish in the course of the twenty-first century is to make even better use of natural products for medicinal purposes. Technology *cannot* replace nature, but it can help us modify and improve natural products not only for medicine but for industry and agriculture as well.

The medicines of the twenty-first century will not come solely from natural sources. Some will be designed from scratch, based on a better comprehension of the human body (and much of that understanding will be based on our having mapped the nervous system by using natural poisons from creatures like cone snails and spiders). Others—like the clot-buster TPA (alteplase) and the new breast cancer drug Herceptin—will be modeled after compounds in the human body (which, therefore, must be considered drugs derived from nature). Additional pharmaceuticals will be produced through semisynthesis: taking a natural compound and modifying the molecule to make it more effective and/or less toxic (as will be the case with anticancer medicines from coral sponges). And other drugs will be identical to products found in nature, but created from scratch in the laboratory to avoid having to harvest the compound from the wild.

As we enter the new century, however, more Americans are visiting "nontraditional" healers than physicians. The sterility, the bureaucracy, the ineffectiveness of Western medicine in treating certain disorders has led people to investigate alternatives. Many of these alternatives—aromatherapy, bee venom therapy, ayurvedic medicine, herbalism—feature natural products as healing tools. The future of Western healing is not alternative medicine—where you visit your family doctor and refrain from telling her or him that an herbalist is also treating you because you fear their reaction. Rather, the future is complementary medicine, which brings together the best of all healing traditions under one roof: from acupuncture to shamanistic hypnotherapy to surgery. And natural products—not only prescription and over-the-counter pharmaceuticals but herbs, vitamins, and other supplements (currently worth twelve billion dollars in retain sales)—will prove to be an integral part of this new healing tradition.

Environmental degradation and destruction remain the major threats to the realization of this scenario. Overpopulation, deforestation, pollution, and the wildlife trade threaten not only the viability of endangered species but also the survival of our own species. If we deprive ourselves of the weapons needed to combat and defeat the diseases that always have threatened us (and always will), we endanger ourselves. Finding the means to both coexist with and benefit from creatures like cone snails, poison dart frogs, leeches, and maggots may often lack appeal in an aesthetic sense but nonetheless will prove invaluable to our own self-interest. Better management of our relationship with the species that share our planet ensures a better life for the future.

SELECTED BIBLIOGRAPHY

Chapter One

Adams, M., and G. Swanson. 1996. "Neurotoxins." *Trends in Neuroscience* (supplement; June).

Angier, N. 1995. "Flyspeck on a lobster lip turns biology on its ear." *New York Times* (Dec. 14), p. A1.

Aregood, C. 1998. "Poisons provide keys to cures." *Sunday News Journal* (Wilmington, Del.; May 10).

Barinaga, M. 1990. "Science digests the secrets of voracious killer snails." *Science* 249: 250–51.

Benyus, J. 1997. *Biomimicry*. New York: Morrow.

Canine, C. 1997. "Pain, profit, and sweet relief." *Worth* (Mar.), pp. 76–82, 151–58.

Chivian, E. 1997. "Global environmental degradation and biodiversity loss: Implications for human health." In *Biodiversity and Human Health* (F. Grifo and J. Rosenthal, eds.). Washington, D.C.: Island.

Cragg, G., D. Newman, and K. Snader. 1997. "Natural products in drug discovery and development." *Journal of Natural Products* 60: 52.

Daly, J. 1995. "Chemistry of poison in amphibian skin." *Proceedings of the National Academy of Sciences* 92: 9–13.

Gibbs, W. 1996. "A new way to spell relief—v-e-n-o-m." *Scientific American* (Feb.), pp. 28–30.

Grifo, F., and J. Rosenthal, eds. 1997. *Biodiversity and Human Health*. Washington, D.C.: Island Press.

Kolata, G. 1996. "Deadly snails take pinpoint aim." *New York Times* (Aug. 6), p. C1.

Miljanich, G. 1997. "Venom peptides as human pharmaceuticals." *Science and Medicine* 4(5): 6–15.

Myers, C., J. Daly, and B. Malkin. 1978. "A dangerously toxic new frog (*Phyllobates*) used by Embera Indians of western Colombia." *Bulletin of the American Museum of Natural History* 161(2): 311–65.

Olivera, B., et al. 1990. "Diversity of *Conus* neuropeptides." *Science* 249: 257–63.

"The pharmaceutical industry." 1998. *The Economist* (Feb. 21), pp. 1–18.

Varmus, H. 1998. "NIH funding increases." *Congressional Testimony* (Mar. 26).

Chapter Two

Brown, M. 1995. "Evolving in the dark." *New York Times* (Dec. 12), p. C1.

Coats, A. 1969. *The Quest for Plants*. London: Studio Vista.

Crystal, D. 1997. "Vanishing languages." *Civilization* (Feb.), pp. 40–45.

"The earth's hidden life." 1996. *The Economist* (Dec. 21), pp. 111–13.

"The eyes have it." 1996. *New Scientist* (July 6), p. 3.

Gould, S. J. 1996. "Life on Mars? So what?" *New York Times* Op-Ed (Aug. 11), p. 13.

Griggs, B. 1981. *Green Pharmacy*. Rochester, Vt.: Healing Arts.

Henahan, S. 1996. "Cave creatures without light." *Access Excellence On-Line*. www.acessexcellence.org.

Huxtable, R. 1992. "The pharmacology of extinction." *Journal of Ethnopharmacology* 37: 1–11.

———. 1995. "Extinction and the loss of phytochemical diversity and pharmacological potential." In *Phytochemicals and Health* (D. Gustine and H. Flores, eds.), pp. 247–59. Rockville, Md.: American Society of Plant Pathologists.

Juma, C. 1989. *The Gene Hunters*. Princeton, N.J.: Princeton University Press.

Lovejoy, T. 1995. "Bugs, plants, and progress." *New York Times* Op-Ed (May 28), p. 29.

Majno, G. 1975. *The Healing Hand*. Cambridge: Harvard University Press.

Moukheiber, Z. 1998. "A hail of silver bullets." *Forbes* (Jan. 26), pp. 76–81.

Pliny. 1991. *Natural History: A Selection*. New York: Penguin.

Radetsky, P. 1998. "Last days of the wonder drugs." *Discover* (June), pp. 76–85.

Riddle, J. 1992. *Contraception and Abortion from the Ancient World to the Renaissance*. Cambridge: Harvard University Press.

Riddle, J., and J. Estes. 1992. "Oral contraceptives in ancient and medieval times." *American Scientist* 80 (3): 226–33.

Tyldesley, J. 1996. *Hatchepsut—The Female Pharoah*. New York: Viking.

Wilson, E. O. 1992. *The Diversity of Life*. Cambridge: Harvard University Press.

Chapter Three

Borel, J., Z. Kis, and T. Beveridge. 1995. "The history of the discovery and development of Cyclosporine." In *The Search for Anti-Inflammatory Drugs* (V. Merluzzi and J. Adas, eds.), pp. 27–63. Boston: Birkhauser.

Burger, A. 1986. *Drugs and People*. Charlottesville: University of Virginia Press.

Coleman, K. 1995. "A magical mold." *World and I* 10 (July 1), p. 166.

Hobbs, C. 1995. *Medicinal Mushrooms*. Santa Cruz, Calif.: Botanica.

Holmes, B. 1996. "Life unlimited." *New Scientist* (Feb. 10), pp. 26–29.

Jacobs, F. 1985. *Breakthrough: The Story of Penicillin*. New York: Dodd, Mead.

Katzung, B., and A. Trevor. 1995. *Pharmacology*. Norwalk, Conn.: Appleton and Lange.

Lemonick, M. 1994. "Revenge of the killer microbes." *Time* (Sept. 12), pp. 60–69.

Levy, S. 1992. *The Antibiotic Paradox*. New York: Plenum.

Preston, R. 1994. *The Hot Zone*. New York: Random House.

Reese, R., and R. Betts. 1993. *Handbook of Antibiotics*. Boston: Little, Brown.

Robbers, J. E., M. K. Speedie, and V. E. Tyler. 1996. *Pharmacognosy and Pharmacobiotechnology*. Baltimore: Williams and Wilkins.

Ryan, F. 1993. *The Forgotten Plague*. Boston: Back Bay Books.

Singleton, P. 1995. *Bacteria*. New York: John Wiley.

Spindler, K. 1994. *The Man in the Ice*. London: Weidenfeld and Nicholson.

Chapter Four

Barinaga, M. 1993. "New test catches drug-resistant TB in the spotlight." *Science* 250: 750.

Beattie, A. 1992. "Discovering new biological resources—chance or reason?" *BioScience* 42(4): 290–92.

———. 1994. "Invertebrates as economic resources." *Memoirs of the Queensland Museum* 36(1): 7–11.

———. 1996. "Putting biodiversity to work." *Search* 27(4): 111–13.

Berenbaum, M. 1995. *Bugs in the System*. Reading, Mass.: Helix Books.

Eisner, T. 1972. "Chemical defense against predation in arthropods." In *Chemical Ecology* (E. Sondheimer and K. Simeone, eds.), pp. 157–217. New York: Academic Press.

Forsyth, A. 1990. *Portraits of the Rainforest*. Toronto: Camden House.

Forsyth, A., and K. Miyata. 1984. *Tropical Nature*. New York: Scribner.

Nabhan, G., and S. Buchmann. 1996. *Forgotten Pollinators*. Washington, D.C.: Island.

Phillips, K. 1991. "Spider man." *Discover* (June 1), pp. 48–53.

Weil, A. 1995. *Spontaneous Healing*. New York: Knopf.

Chapter Five

Bisset, N. 1991. "One man's poison, another man's medicine?" *Journal of Ethnopharmacology* 32: 71–81.

Fields, W. 1991. "The history of leeching and hirudin." *Haemostasis* 21, supplement 1: 3–10.

Krezel, A., G. Wagner, J. Seymour-Ulmer, and R. Lazarus. 1994. "Structure of decorsin." *Science* 264: 1944–47.

Lent, C. 1986. "Medical and scientific uses of the leech." *Nature* 323: 494.

Root-Bernstein, R. and M. 1997. *Honey, Mud, and Maggots*. Boston: Houghton-Mifflin.

Rundle, R. 1996. "Bats and ticks hold clues to new drugs." *Wall Street Journal* (Apr. 16), pp. B1, B6.

Sawyer, R. 1986. *Leech Biology and Behavior*. Oxford: Clarendon.

———. 1991. "In search of the giant Amazon leech." *Smithsonian* (Dec.), pp. 66–67.

Chapter Six

Amato, I. 1992. "From hunter magic, a pharmacopeia?" *Science* 258: 1306.

Bevin, C., and M. Zasloff. 1990. "Peptides from frog skins." *Annual Review of Biochemistry* 59: 395–414.

Bishop, J. 1980. "Stalking a killer." *Wall Street Journal* (June 6), p. A1.

Cushman, D., H. Cheung, E. Sabo, and M. Ondetti. 1982. "Development and design of specific inhibitors of angiotensin-converting enzyme." *American Journal of Cardiology* 49(6): 1390–94.

Daly, J. 1995. "Alkaloids from frog skins." *Brazilian Journal of Medical and Biological Research* 28: 1033–42.

Glausiusz, J. 1998. "The frog solution." *Discover* (June), pp. 88–94.

Gorman, P. 1990. "People of the jaguar." *Shaman's Drum* (Fall), pp. 40–49.

————. 1995. "Between the canopy and the forest floor." *High Times* (Jan.), pp. 44–47, 66–67.

Grenard, S. 1994. *Medical Herpetology.* Pottsville, Pa.: Reptile and Amphibian Magazine.

Griffiths, V. 1998. "Venom may slow speed of cancer." *Denver Rocky Mountain News* (Aug. 27), p. 40A.

McKean, K. 1986. "Pain." *Discover* (Oct.), pp. 82–92.

Popescu, P. 1991. *Amazon Beaming.* New York: Penguin.

Zasloff, M. 1987. "Magainins." *Proceedings of the National Academy of Sciences* 84 (Aug.): 5449–53.

Chapter Seven

Broad, W. 1997. *The Universe Below.* New York: Simon and Schuster.

Carte, B. 1996. "Biomedical potential of marine natural products." *Bio-Science* 46(4): 271–86.

Der Marderosian, A., and L. Liberti. 1988. *Natural Product Medicine.* Philadelphia: G. F. Stickley.

Halstead, B. 1992. *Dangerous Aquatic Animals of the World.* Princeton, N.J.: Darwin.

Kreig, M. 1964. *Green Medicine.* Chicago: Rand McNally.

Sargent, W. 1987. *The Year of the Crab.* New York: Norton.

Van Dover, C. 1996. *The Octopus' Garden.* Reading, Mass.: Helix Books.

Chapter Eight

Acosta, W. 1996. *Bombardier Beetles and Fever Trees.* Reading Mass.: Helix Books.

Biser, J. 1998. "Really wild remedies." *Zoogoer* (Jan.–Feb.), pp. 7–15.

Cowen, R. 1990. "Medicine on the wild side." *Science News* 138: 280–82.

Janzen, J. 1978. "Complications in interpreting the chemical defenses of trees against tropical arboreal plant-eating vertebrates." In *The Ecology of Arboreal Folivores* (G. Montgomery, ed.), pp. 73–84. Washington, D.C.: Smithsonian Institution Press.

Link, K. 1959. "The discovery of dicumerol and its sequels." *Circulation* 19: 97–107.

McRae, M. 1994. "Creature cures." *Equinox* 75: 47–55.

Montgomery, S. 1991. *Walking with the Great Apes.* Boston: Houghton-Mifflin.

Chapter Nine

Balick, M., and P. Cox. 1996. *Plants, People, and Culture*. New York: Scientific American Library.

Campbell, J. 1987. *Primitive Mythology*. New York: Penguin.

Clottes, J., and D. Lewis-Williams. 1996. *The Shamans of Prehistory*. New York: Harry Abrams.

Eliade, M. 1964. *Shamanism*. Princeton, N.J.: Princeton University Press.

LaBarre, W. 1972. "Hallucinogens and the shamanic origins of religion." In *Flesh of the Gods* (P. Furst, ed.), pp. 261–78. London: Allen and Unwin.

Mann, J. 1994. *Murder, Magic, and Medicine*. Oxford: Oxford University Press.

Ortiz de Montellano, B. 1990. *Aztec Medicine, Health, and Nutrition*. New Brunswick, N.J.: Rutgers University Press.

Plotkin, M. 1994. *Tales of a Shaman's Apprentice*. New York: Penguin.

Prance, G., W. Balee, B. Boom, and R. Carneiro. 1987. "Quantitative ethnobotany and the case for conservation in Amazonia." *Conservation Biology* 1: 296–310.

Schultes, R. E., and A. Hofmann. 1979. *Plants of the Gods*. New York: McGraw-Hill.

Solecki, R. S. 1975. "Shanidar IV." *Science* 190: 880–81.

Torrey, F. 1984. *Witchdoctors and Psychiatrists*. Northvale, N.J.: J. Aronson.

Vitebsky, P. 1995. *The Shaman*. Boston: Little, Brown.

Vogel, V. 1970. *American Indian Medicine*. Norman, Okla.: University of Oklahoma Press.

INDEX

Abbott Laboratories, 6, 162
ABT-594, 6, 16, 162
ACE (angiotensin-converting enzyme), 127–28
acetylsalicylic acid, 28
actinomycetes, 51
adenine arabinoside (ara-A), 147
adolapin, 87
Aggrastat (tirofiban), 129, 130, 131, 132
agonists, 9
aguardiente, 182
AIDS, 30, 64–65, 147–48
ajmaline, 156
algae, 49; blue-green, 28–29, 140, 151–52, 172
Ali, Karriem, 30
alkaloids, 29, 196
alteplase (TPA), 207
alternative medicines, 26–27, 207
Alzheimer's disease, 6
Amazon:
  aerial mapping of, 35
  Gorman in, 117–19
  habitat destruction in, 155–56, 180
  McIntyre in, 115–17
  Maroons in, 168–69, 172
  medical legacy of, 155–57
  shamans in, 117–23, 179–87, 190
amphibians:
  antibiotics from, 67–68
  extinction of, 132–33
  frogs, 3–6, 115, 120–23, 161–62
analgesics (painkillers), 10, 144
ancrod (Arvin), 130–31

anesthesia, 27
anesthetics, 121
angina, 102, 129–30
animal familiars, 198–99
antagonists, 9
antiamoebic properties, 165
antiarrhythmics, 121
antibiotics:
  from bacteria, 51, 66–68
  drug-resistant, 30, 62–64, 67
  effectiveness of, 61
  in foods, 64, 67
  function of, 55
  from insects, 90–91
  from jungle plants, 162, 165
  me-too drugs, 66
  as miracle drugs, 62–63
  new sources of, 66–68
  penicillin, 47, 54–60, 61
  from sea creatures, 143–44
  synthetic, 57*n*
  use of term, 25–26
  wartime uses of, 53–54, 57–58, 60
anticoagulants, 99–104, 108, 111–12, 128–31, 159–60
anticonvulsants, 121
antidiarrheal preparations, 170
antidysentery drugs, 157
antihypertension drugs, 128
anti-inflammatories, 87, 143–44
antimelanomas, 161
antimicrobial compounds, 157
antiplaque agents, 200
antistatin, 104
antivirals, 140, 147
antiworm properties, 162, 165, 170

ants:
    antibiotics from, 85
    for arthritis, 71–72
    spiders as mimics of, 81
    wounds stitched by, 84–85
apamin, 87
apes:
    DNA of, 169–70
    plants used by, 162–66, 170
apitherapy, 88
ara-A (adenine arabinoside), 147
ara-C (cytosine arabinoside), 146
arecoline, 166
arrow poisons, 108–12, 120
arteries, reconnection of, 105–6
arthritis, 71–73
    ant venoms for, 71–72
    bee venoms for, 86, 87–88
    leeches and, 104
artifact of collection, 170
Arvin (ancrod), 130–31
Asclepius, 124
aspen bark, 171
Aspilia daisy, 162, 163
aspirin, 9, 27, 28
assassin beetles, 46, 78
ayahuasca ritual, 180–86, 188–89,
    196, 202
AZT (azidothymidine), 47, 148

bacteria, 49–52
    antibiotics from, 51, 66–68
    classification of, 50
    diseases caused by, 50–51
    drug-resistant, 30, 62–67, 90–91
    flesh-eating, 65–66
    in hospitals, 64–65
    new species of, 52, 65
    plasmids to, 65
    reproduction of, 63–64
Baer, William, 108
bald eagles, 174–75
barbamide, 152
batrachotoxin, 121
Batzella sponges, 148

bears, 24, 171
Beattie, Andrew J., 84–85
bedbugs, 76–77
bee pollen, 88
bees, 85–90, 91
beeswax, 88
beetles, 77–79
Benyus, Jeannine, 23
benzene, 198
Beraldo, Wilson, 127
Berenbaum, May, 74, 76
Bergmann, W., 146–47, 148
betel palm, 166
biodiversity, 31, 37, 39, 73–74, 103,
    146
biomimicry, 22–23
bioprospecting, history of, 24
biorational deduction, 84–85
biotechnology, 27
birds, plants used by, 172–75
black bile, as "humor," 97
blister beetles, 78–79
blood:
    functions of, 99
    as "humor," 97
blood clot–busters, 104, 129, 207
blood clotting, 99–102, 105, 131
bloodletting, 97–99
blood pressure, 126
bloodroot plants, 200
bloodsuckers, 104–5; *see also*
    leeches
blood thinners, 99
blowflies, maggots of, 107
blue-green algae, 28–29, 140,
    151–52, 172
Bobbitt, John, 106
boldo shrub, 195
Bolivian hemorrhagic fever, 63
bone, synthetic, 150
Botox, 8
Bouchard, Lucien, 66
BPH (benign prostate enlarge-
    ment), 200
bradykinin, 127